Molecular Histopathology and Cytopathology

Edited by Adem Kara, Volkan Gelen and Hülya Kara

Published in London, United Kingdom

Molecular Histopathology and Cytopathology
http://dx.doi.org/10.5772/intechopen.105300
Edited by Adem Kara, Volkan Gelen and Hülya Kara

Contributors
Dyah Oktavianie Ayu Pratama, Arni Kusuma Dewi, Widjiati Widjiati, Bambang Purwanto, Dang Viet Duc, Nguyen Thanh Huy, Tran Quoc Quy, Nguyen Tat Tho, Shivani Gandhi, Ishani Gupta, Reetika Menia, Raman Kumar, Safiya Tazeen, Mohammed Ibrahim, Maisun Mohamed Al-Zorgani, Hassan Ugail, Klaus Pors, Abdullahi Magaji Dauda, Flora Thanadar Ajmiree, Marijana Popović Bajić, Vanja Opačić Galić, Violeta Petrović, Smiljana Paraš, Vukoman Jokanović, Slavoljub Živković, Natsuko Mizutani, Adem Kara, Volkan Gelen, Hülya Kara

First published in London, United Kingdom, 2023 by IntechOpen
IntechOpen is the global imprint of INTECHOPEN LIMITED, registered in England and Wales, registration number: 11086078, 5 Princes Gate Court, London, SW7 2QJ, United Kingdom

British Library Cataloguing-in-Publication Data
A catalogue record for this book is available from the British Library

Additional hard and PDF copies can be obtained from orders@intechopen.com

Molecular Histopathology and Cytopathology
Edited by Adem Kara, Volkan Gelen and Hülya Kara
p. cm.
Print ISBN 978-1-83768-643-8
Online ISBN 978-1-83768-644-5
eBook (PDF) ISBN 978-1-83768-645-2

For EU product safety concerns:
IN TECH d.o.o., Prolaz Marije Krucifikse Kozulić 3, 51000 Rijeka, Croatia,
info@intechopen.com or visit our website at intechopen.com.

Meet the editors

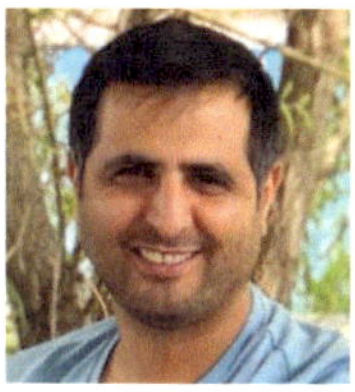

Dr. Kara completed his doctorate in the Department of Histology and Embryology at the Faculty of Medicine in 2012. He worked as a lecturer in the Faculty of Veterinary Medicine, Department of Histology and Embryology, Atatürk University, Bingöl Universities, Turkey. Dr. Kara has authored and co-authored fifty-seven journal papers, four book chapters, and thirty other types of publications.

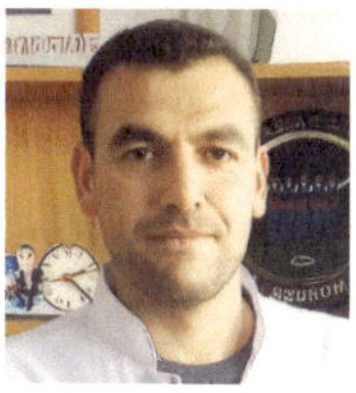

Dr. Gelen is a physiology specialist who received his veterinary degree from Kafkas University, Turkey, in 2011. From 2011 to 2015, he worked as an assistant in the Department of Physiology, Faculty of Veterinary Medicine, Atatürk University, Turkey. In 2016, he joined Kafkas University as an assistant professor where he has been engaged in various academic activities. Dr. Gelen has sixty journal articles and twenty poster presentations to his credit. His research interests include physiology, the endocrine system, cancer, diabetes, cardiovascular diseases, and isolated organ bath system studies.

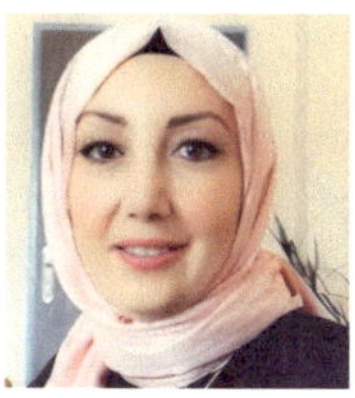

Dr. Kara completed her doctorate in the Department of Anatomy at the Faculty of Veterinary Medicine in 2017. She became an associate professor in 2022 and is currently working in the Faculty of Veterinary Medicine, Department of Anatomy, Atatürk University, Turkey. She has authored and co-authored nineteen journal papers, two book chapters, and thirty-two other types of publications.

Contents

Preface

This book presents some topics in histopathology and cytopathology that may interest histopathologists and other professionals interested in pathology. Histopathology and cytopathology use fundamental knowledge from the biological and anatomical sciences to diagnose and determine the severity and progression of a condition and evaluate the possible response to certain treatments. It is an expanding discipline with new technologies and histopathological methods regularly being developed. Chapters in this book cover topics that illustrate the various perspectives involved in histopathology and cytopathology.

Adem Kara Ph.D.
Faculty of Science,
Department of Molecular Biology and Genetics,
Erzurum Technical University,
Erzurum, Turkey

Volkan Gelen Ph.D.
Faculty of Veterinary Medicine,
Department of Physiology,
Kafkas University,
Kars, Turkey

Hülya Kara Ph.D.
Faculty of Veterinary Medicine,
Department of Anatomy,
Atatürk University,
Erzurum, Turkey

Section 1

Molecular Histopathology

Chapter 1

Introduction of Histopathology

Arni Kusuma Dewi, Bambang Purwanto and Widjiati

Abstract

Histopathology is the science that studies disease pathology through morphological changes that can be seen microscopically. The word histopathology was first known to be introduced in a book entitled "On the Nature and Structure Characteristic of Cancer" by Johannes Muller in 1838. Before histopathology, doctors distinguished diseases based on macroscopically visible morphology organ changes (anatomy) in the operating room or during forensic autopsies. However, this expertise requires another diagnosis method to ensure that several differential diagnoses indicate the same anatomical morphological changes. Definitive diagnosis is obtained by taking a small organ tissue sample during surgery (biopsy), which is then viewed microscopically. This diagnosis method is called histopathological diagnosis. For example, a person with hearing loss has received a differential diagnosis of conduction or sensorineural hearing loss. An external macroscopic physical examination for this patient is as necessary as internal imaging. The condition's pathological cause can be ascertained by additional histopathology biopsies. However, invasive histopathology procedures can be uncomfortable and cause harm. Histopathology for diagnostic or research purposes requires two fundamental things: the microscope as a tool and the development of histopathological techniques.

Keywords: histopathology, diagnose, research, biopsy, surgery

1. Introduction

Histopathology is very widely used, not only as a diagnostic tool but also as an examination tool, monitoring the effects of therapy or estimating a disease's prognosis. Microscopes are necessary equipment for carrying out histopathological functions. Histopathological preparations rely on microscopes, as does result examination [1].

A microscope is a tool for viewing cell and tissue structures that cannot be seen by the naked eye because of their micron or smaller size. The cell is the smallest unit of life. Several cells that come together and perform the same function are referred to as tissue. Organs are several tissues that come together and form the same function. The microscope was first introduced by Zacharias Jansen and his father in 1591 [2], and it was then perfected by Leeuwenhoek in 1673. Furthermore, along with the need to see certain tissue structures, microscopes evolved from light to fluorescence microscopes [2].

Histopathology is a technique for making histological preparations for diseased tissues. These techniques include fixation techniques, tissue processing, tissue sectioning, and tissue staining. Fixation techniques are needed for hardening, keeping the cell death process from continuing, and keeping structural molecules from being damaged. Tissue processing aims to remove water from the intracell and replace it with a medium that can harden the cell structure to make it easy to cut. Tissue sectioning refers to cutting the prepared specimen into several slices. Finally, tissue staining aims to color the cell and tissue structures with specific staining according to the examination's purpose [3].

Microscopy and histopathology technique development are fundamental things to know when making examination preparations and reading tissue preparations from appropriate controls to ensure good examination quality [4].

2. Microscope development

A microscope is a tool used to view tissues and organs' microscopic structures. Microscopes work the same way eyes work. Light, which is an electromagnetic spectrum, is transmitted to the cornea and through the eye's diaphragm (pupil) until it reaches the retina. Whereas in light microscopes, the light that hits the specimen preparation is transmitted by the microscope diaphragm and then captured by the objective and ocular lens for the eye. The resulting image's magnification depends on the objective and ocular lenses' sizes [2]. The following are the microscopes commonly used for a histopathology examination.

2.1 Light microscopy

Early in the sixteenth century, the first microscope was assembled by Jansen and his father. It used the light from the sun (**Figure 1**). The scientists at that time did not feel comfortable using this microscope because the light source did not fall on one point, thus interfering with the view. Sun or white light consists of several color spectrums. When it falls on a simple lens like Jansen's work, it will make the colors scatter according to their wavelength. This is known as chromatic aberration. This became the basis for Leeuwenhoek in 1673 to make two lenses with different mediums. Colors that degraded due to certain wavelengths could be absorbed by the lens medium. The achromatic is a lens medium that can correct two spectrums of blue and red, while an apochromat medium is a lens medium that corrects two spectrums of green and yellow [2, 3]. Leeuwenhoek's microscope can magnify a maximum of 300 times the resulting image. At the time, he could identify bacteria, muscles, teeth, and blood cells [3]. The microscope's components were then developed to correct chromatic aberration with the discovery of lens mediums that fit examination needs. Leeuwenhoek's principal work was the basic development of the light microscope (**Figure 2**).

Light microscopes' components and models evolve with their needs and uses. Currently, apart from being a diagnostic tool, light microscopes are also used for teaching and learning purposes. Several types of microscopes have been established with their respective advantages for teaching purposes. The double or triple ocular lens and light microscope models that are connected to the computer with or without application are widely used. **Figure 3** shows the resulting image with a light microscope.

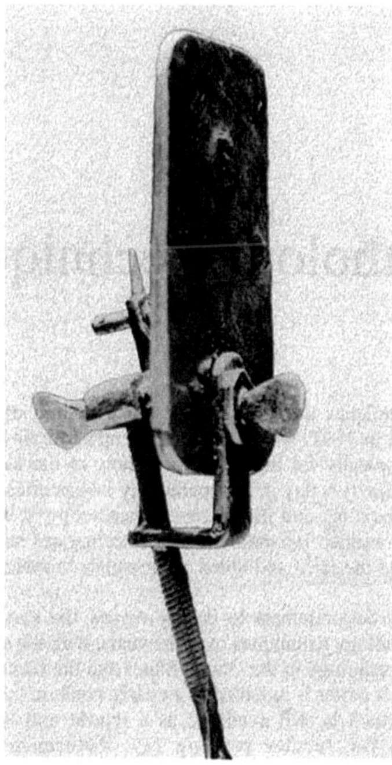

Figure 1.
Jansen's microscope with the single lens source [2].

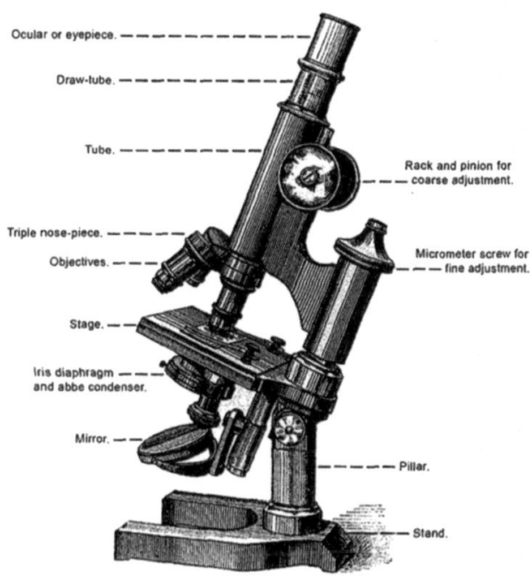

Figure 2.
Light microscopy model in general source [2].

2.2 Electron microscopy

The electron microscope was first assembled by Ernst Ruska in 1920. This microscope's purpose is to view biological ultrastructures and identify diseases that are difficult to explain. Its working principle is to use light with short wavelengths

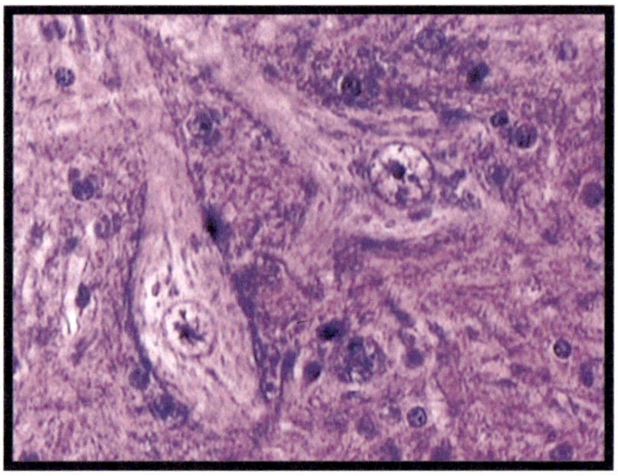

Figure 3.
Image of the spinal cord by light microscope with 400 times magnification.

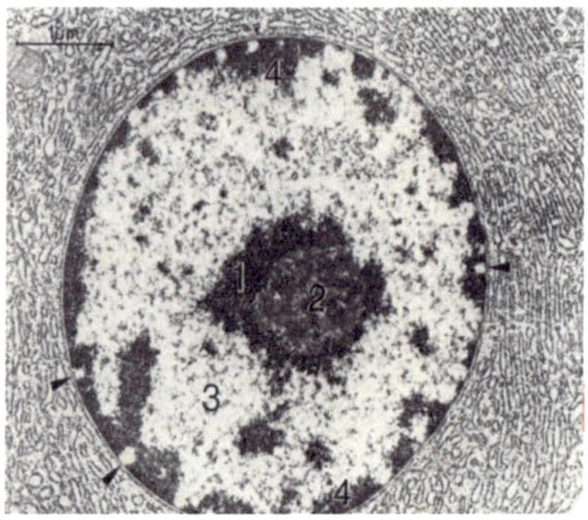

Figure 4.
Image of nucleus and RER neuron cell by TEM.

to produce better resolution and magnification. Resolution is the ratio between the wavelength and the width of the diaphragm opening [3, 5].

The types of electron microscopes are the scanning electron microscope (SEM), the transmission electron microscope (TEM), and the cryo-electron microscope (Cryo-EM) [5–7]. SEM is a type of electron microscope that can only take ultrasound images on surfaces, such as the skin's epidermal layer. TEM is a type of electron microscope that can take ultra-cell images of cytoplasmic organelles such as mitochondria and rough endoplasmic reticulum (RER). Cryo-EM is a type of electron microscope that can produce ultra-cell images up to atoms in 3D for single particle analysis, such as on certain proteins, with better resolution [5–7].

The difference in preparation between a light microscope and SEM or TEM is that the specimen's maximum size before processing is cut at 1 mm^3 as well as its fixative medium, which will be discussed in detail in topic 3 [3]. The differences in preparation between the light microscope and Cryo-EM are specimen screening and preparation, data acquisition, image processing, and structure validation [6]. **Figure 4** shows an image result from EM.

2.3 Phase contrast microscopy/interference microscopy

The working principle of a phase-contrast microscope or interference microscope is that the light is blocked by the specimen, thus producing a "halo" in the resulting image. A halo pattern will form on the bright and dark bands when light passes through the specimen. Besides the halo, the resulting image is also a color gradation and a quantitative index of refraction. This microscope shows biological structures in larger pieces than other types of microscopes [3].

2.4 Fluorescence microscopy

Fluorescence is light that is reflected by objects or specimens that are lit at a certain wavelength. Objects or specimens that can emit fluorescence alone are called fluorophores, also called primary fluorescence or autofluorescence. Some examples are porphyria, elastic fiber, collagen, vitamin A, and lipofuscin [3].

Specimen fluorescence can also be induced by adding a substance, such as a certain antibody painted with a fluorescence agent like blue, green, or ultraviolet fluorochrome [2]. This was first introduced by Coons, Creech, and Jones in 1941.

Fluorescence microscopy's development from two dimensions (2D) to three dimensions (3D) makes pathological models in biological tissues clearer. In 3D fluorescence microscopy, axial scanning is required for several specimen pieces that make up the volume. Data is transferred to a computer with certain applications. The required variables can be calculated quantitatively or only qualitatively [8]. This microscope's weakness is that the entire field of view will show fluorochrome, including areas that are not the focus of research [3]. This weakness became the basis for confocal microscopy development.

2.5 Confocal microscopy

Confocal microscopy enhances the image results from fluorescence microscopy. Confocal microscopes have a pinhole component to only focus the image on the part being examined. Microscopic imaging results can be seen at one time [3].

Histopathology has an important role in the diagnosis. However, ordinary histological techniques after a biopsy are not able to describe details such as the boundaries of cancer cell development that must be taken during the operation at the same time (during surgery). To overcome this, the confocal microscope technique was developed into confocal laser endomicroscopy (CLE). The CLE technique greatly improves the surgical outcome and prognosis of most cancers [8].

The CLE technique requires intravenous injection of fluorosphere contrast enhancer before surgery begins. Sodium fluorescence (SF) is a type of fluorosphere that has been studied. It has a composition of 5 mL in 10% saline solution and must be injected just before surgery. The second type is 5-aminolevulinic acid (5-ALA) with a composition of 20 mg/kg, which is injected 3 hours before surgery. The time of contrast enhancer administration from seven studies gave different results in terms of cell contour [8].

Pathological feature observation results using the CLE technique were better than those with ordinary histological techniques. The contour cells could be differentiated in terms of vascular proliferation, cellular density, and irregular cell phenotype

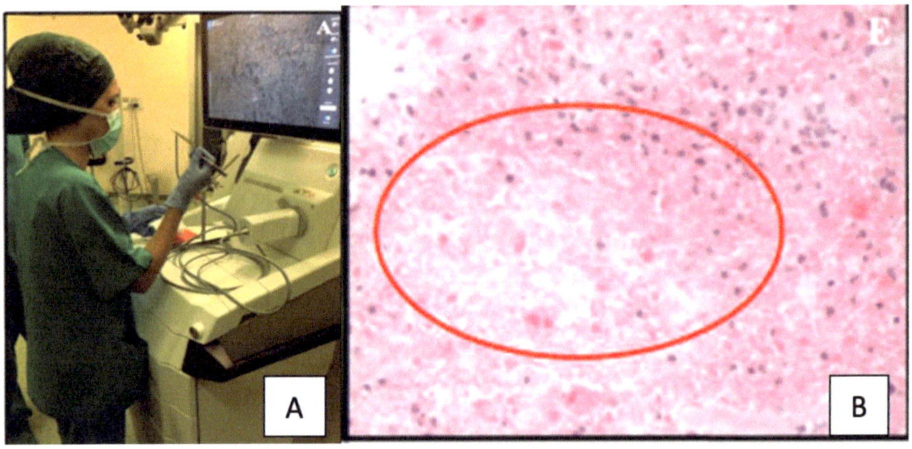

Figure 5.
A. Confocal imaging of CLE during operation. B. Convivo ex vivo CLE image that show low cellular density (red circle). Source [8].

between high-grade gliomas, low-grade gliomas, and normal glia at the same time during surgery. Based on research, the imaging results were better when using SF to show the cells' contours (**Figure 5**) [8].

3. Histopathology technique development

Histopathology techniques refer to procedures that must be carried out to produce histological preparations of diseased tissue which will be analyzed visually. These techniques include 10% formalin buffer fixation, embedded paraffin, manual sectioning, dewaxed sectioning, routine staining with Hematoxylin–Eosin (HE), or special staining such as immunohistochemistry (IHC), in situ hybridization (ISH), or special staining for connecting tissue [3, 9].

Observations with histopathological techniques are observations done under a light microscope. Imaging evaluations are generated by comparing diseased tissue with control or healthy tissue [9]. The purpose of this evaluation is to help diagnose, plan therapy, and predict a disease's prognosis [10].

This histopathology technique, which has been practiced since 1970, can only be partially done automatically. The embedding and sectioning processes must be done manually [9]. Several new procedures have been developed to improve image quality from conventional histopathological techniques, such as fixation procedures to protect RNA from autolysis damage during the death process [10].

3.1 Fixation

Fixation is the initial procedure after a fresh specimen is taken during surgery. The purpose of fixation is to prevent the autolysis process and postmortem cell death, which can affect water, electrolytes, and enzyme activity dynamics. If the autolysis process and cell death are not prevented, then the cells or tissues in the specimen will become easily overgrown with microorganisms [9].

Fixation methods are typically either physical or chemical. The physical method, for example, involves packing specimens cut during operations in vacuum plastic bags and storing them at 4°C. This method can protect RNA and prevent dehydration and enzyme autolysis. The chemical method is done by immersing the specimen in a chemical solution [3].

Chemical solutions that are routinely used are neutral buffered formalin 10% (NBF 10%) or Formalin-Fixed Paraffin-Embedded (FFPE), glutaraldehyde, mixed formaldehyde, and glutaraldehyde solution, and osmium tetraoxide. NBF 10% or FFPE is used routinely for specimens viewed under the light microscope. Meanwhile, glutaraldehyde, or a mixture of formaldehyde and glutaraldehyde and osmium tetraoxide is used routinely for specimens viewed under an electron microscope [3, 11]. Alcohol can also be used for fixation, but it is necessary to pay attention to its percentage and fixation time. This is because alcohol attracts water very quickly and denatures proteins. Research conducted by Arni et al. states that alcohol fixation can be done with ethanol with gradual concentrations, from 40% for 24 hours and up to 60% within the next 24 hours. The results of this study showed a good contour cell seen in the light microscope [11].

Neutral buffered formalin 10% (NBF 10%), paraformaldehyde 4%, and formalin are aldehyde groups. NBF 10%, paraformaldehyde 4% is a fixation medium that is routinely used by pathologists. Formaldehyde is a gas that dissolves in water to form methylene hydrate. Formalin is formed from 37 **to** 40% formaldehyde and 60–63% water. This process can take days if plain water is used to dissolve the formaldehyde. This is different if it is dissolved in a buffer solution at physiological pH. This fixation solution is known as neutral buffered formalin 10%. NBF 10% is enriched with 10% methanol to prevent precipitation to paraformaldehyde. Paraformaldehyde dissolved in water and containing 1% methanol is called 4% paraformaldehyde. NBF 10% is routinely used by pathologists to examine diseased tissue under a light microscope, while 4% paraformaldehyde is used in electron microscopes [12].

The aldehyde group can bond with nitrogen and several protein atoms or adjacent atoms to form a cross-link called a methylene bridge. Tissue reaction to formalin can occur within 24 hours. However, cross-links may weaken the longer the fixation process takes. The cross-links protect the proteins, carbohydrates, and lipids, which are trapped in and not chemically changed. However, if the fixation is carried out for several weeks, the cross-links will be reversible and break the carbohydrates, proteins, and fats' properties [3, 12].

Glutaraldehyde is a small molecule that has two aldehyde groups. Because of this, glutaraldehyde has greater potential to cross-link and is faster than formalin [12]. This protects the ultrastructural components. The cross-link reaction is irreversible. Due to the nature of glutaraldehyde, this fixation medium was used as the first fixation medium for electron microscopy specimen preparations. However, this fixation medium has a weakness when used for special immunohistochemical staining. Because the cross-link reaction is irreversible, staining antibodies cannot enter and allow background staining to occur [3].

Osmium tetraoxide was the first fixation medium for electron microscopy specimen preparation. This fixation medium protects cell and tissue structures that contain lipids and can react to form cross-links on hydrophilic or hydrophobic atoms. However, because of its expense and toxicity, osmium tetraoxide is occasionally used for the second medium fixation instead [3, 12].

3.2 Tissue processing

Tissue processing is a procedure for immersing tissue specimens into paraffin. This aims to make the tissue harder, making it easier to cut thinly. The tool for this procedure is a tissue processor [2, 3]. The tissue processor has a jar or tube consisting of glass or copper which contains 96% alcohol, absolute alcohol, chloroform, chloroform saturated with paraffin, paraffin bath, and water. The jar containing the liquid paraffin is made of heated copper. Tissue processing and embedding last about 26–100 hours or several days. The following is the time needed to produce network embedding with optimal results [2]:

Alcohol 96% 6–24 hours
Alcohol absolute 6–24 hours
Chloroform 6–24 hours
Chloroform saturated with paraffin 6–24 hours
Paraffin bath 2–4 hours
Cool water (quickly).

3.3 Sectioning

Sectioning is a procedure for cutting tissue that has been embedded with paraffin (paraffin block) into several ribbons. Cutting is done using a tool called the microtome. Thickness is generally 3–5 micrometers, except for neural networks, for which optimal results (not too thick) are around 7 micrometers [3, 9].

The ribbon that is formed is put in warm water at a temperature of about 45°C. This pulls and thins the ribbon, allowing it to stretch without bending. It can then be easily positioned on the glass slide. Previously, the glass slides should have been labeled and given glue made from egg whites. After the ribbon is attached, the glass slide is dried at room temperature or heated at room temperature at 37°C [3, 9].

3.4 Staining

A staining procedure is required to be able to evaluate the resulting image under a light microscope. This is because the prepared specimens produced from paraffinization have low contrast. This makes it difficult to distinguish structures [9].

Sectioning, followed by staining, previously had to go through a rehydration stage with xylene as well as absolute alcohol with up to 95% alcohol. This rehydration stage aims to pull out the paraffin from the intracell and the extracellular and replace it with water. This is done because routine dye stains are water-soluble [9].

The following are some of the dyes that are often used by pathologists: Hematoxylin–eosin (HE) stain, osmic acid stain, periodic-acid Schiff (PAS) stain, Masson-Mallory trichrome, and Giemsa [13]. He is the oldest routine stain and is still used as a routine stain by pathologists. There has been an emergence of histopathological dye development because, since 1903, several researchers considered HE staining inadequate. These researchers are M. Heidenhain (1903), Masson (1923), Langeron (1925), and Gabe (1969). They assumed this because no new structures were found when only relying on HE staining. Currently, in addition to staining for specific cell parts, staining techniques have been developed molecularly with immunohistochemistry, immunofluorescence, and in situ hybridization [3, 13].

Osmic acid is used to color fat produced by cells. An example is myelin, which is a glial cell produced by Schwan cells in the peripheral nervous system. PAS staining is used for cells that produce glucose, causing a pink granule to appear in the cytoplasm. The Masson Mallory trichome stain is used to differentiate collagen fibers in several connective tissues. Giemsa is used to stain blood cells for the cytoplasmic granules to be differentiated [13].

Hematoxylin can be found in the inner part of the logwood tree, which was originally found in Central America. Presently, it is grown in the Caribbean islands, Australia, India, Malaysia, and West Africa [14]. When dissolved, hematoxylin contains one or more aluminum-hematein complex cations known as hemalum. Hemalum has a bond with acids, producing a blue or purple color in the nucleus and nuclei. Cations will react with DNA and rRNA in the nucleus [9, 13, 15]. Meanwhile, eosin is a solution that binds to structures other than acids in the cytoplasm and gives it a red color [15].

Hematoxylin is currently scarce, which is why preventive measures are being taken by using substitutes that have the same properties. Substitutes have to be cationic and able to bind to acids. Some of the substitute materials studied are the thiazine, anthocyanin, and anthocyanidins groups. Toluidine blue is a member of the thiazine group. It is used by dissolving it in water until the pH reaches 3–4 or unbuffered. This toluidine blue solution can stain the cell nucleus and sulfated glycosaminoglycans. Sulfated glycosaminoglycans include bony matrix, mast cell granules, and mucous-producing cells. Meanwhile, anthocyanins and anthocyanidins are dyes produced by flowers and fruits, such as Rosella extract and some others that contain flavonoids. The extract is taken by heating it in water with an acidic pH to remove carbohydrates or sugars. The addition of metal salts such as aluminum potassium sulfate (alum) can increase the stain's intensity (**Figure 6**) [14].

3.5 Mounting

Mounting is the last procedure after the coloring process. The staining process is followed by blocking the specimen, making it unable to accept water or other solutions and thereby last a long time. This process begins with cleaning the remaining paint with running water, adding graded alcohol from absolute alcohol to 95% alcohol, then cleaning with xylene [3, 9, 15].

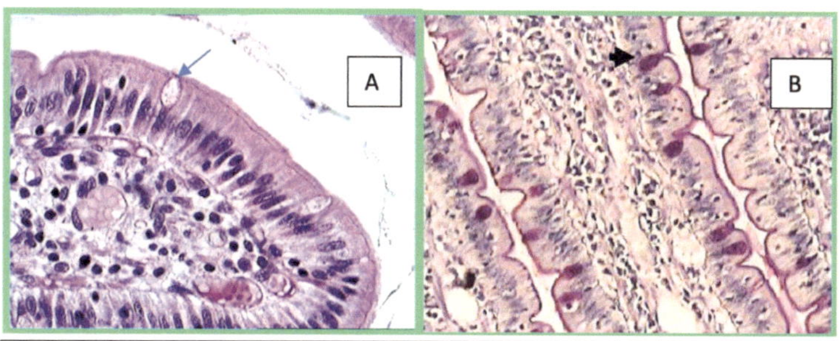

Figure 6.
Villi intestinalis with 400 magnification. A = HE staining intestinalis. The goblet cell cytoplasm looks empty (long arrow). B=PAS staining. The goblet cell cytoplasm looks pink or purple (small arrow).

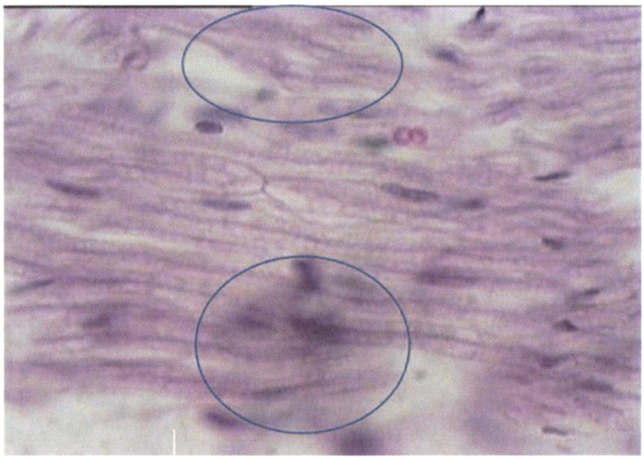

Figure 7.
Peripheral nervous system with 400 magnification. Blue circle shows artifact shadow because of difference of thickness section.

Mounting is done immediately after cleaning with xylene. The specimen preparation is covered with a cover glass with a waterproof adhesive. After that, the evaluation process is carried out under a microscope. Visible cell structure and contour, artifacts, and any color ingredients that did not enter are evaluated [3, 9, 15].

3.6 Artifacts

Artifacts are errors in performing histopathological procedures or techniques. Several types of artifacts can be found. Broken tissue can be caused by tissue being too hard, or the microtome blade needing replacement. Shadow images in the microscope can be caused by different cutting thicknesses. Folded tissue can arise after sectioning if the tissue is not stretched in warm water. Inconsistent staining thickness or out-of-place paint drops can be caused by mishandling the process of cleaning paint with running water (**Figure** 7) [3, 9, 15].

4. Conclusions

Histopathology is basic knowledge for a pathologist. Making a definite diagnosis, planning therapy, and predicting the prognosis of patients' diseases are very dependent on changes in their macroscopic and microscopic structures. These two structural changes are sometimes incompatible because macroscopic changes are preceded by microscopic changes, either due to internal or external stressors. Histopathological evaluation can be done if the imaging obtained is good enough. This is related to the histopathological technique and the type of microscope used.

Acknowledgements

Thank you to the head of the Faculty of Vocational Studies, Universitas Airlangga, who provided support in receiving the invitation to write for IntechOpen. Gratitude is also extended to the head of the Ph.D. program of the Faculty of Medicine,

Universitas Airlangga, who gave his appreciation to those involved in writing these chapters and allowed them to be used for assessment points.

Conflict of interest

The authors declare there was no conflict of interest.

Appendices and nomenclature

5-ALA	5-aminolevulinic acid
CLE	confocal laser endomicroscopy
Cryo-EM	cryo electron microscope
DNA	deoxyribonucleic acid
FFPE	formalin fixed paraffin embedded
HE	hematoxylin – eosin
IHC	immunohistochemistry
ISH	in situ hybridization
NBF	normal buffered formalin
PAS	periodic-acid Schiff
RER	rough endoplasmic reticulum
RNA	ribonucleic acid
SEM	scanning electron microscope
SF	sodium fluorescence
TEM	transmission electron microscope

Author details

Arni Kusuma Dewi, Bambang Purwanto and Widjiati*
Universitas Airlangga, Surabaya, Indonesia

*Address all correspondence to: widjiati@fkh.unair.ac.id

References

[1] Press OA, Guzman R, Cervantes M, Santiago A, Press MF. Characterization of HER2 status by fluorescence in situ hybridization (FISH) and Immunohistochemistry (IHC). Methods in Molecular Biology. 2014;**1180**:181-207

[2] Titford M. A short history of histopathology technique. Journal of Histotechnology. 2006;**29**(2):99-110

[3] Bancroft JD, Gamble M, editors. Theory and Practice Histological Techniques. sixth ed. China: Elsevier; 2008

[4] Montero Llopis P, Senft RA, Ross-Elliott TJ, Stephansky R, Keeley DP, Koshar P, et al. Best practices and tools for reporting reproducible fluorescence microscopy methods. Nature Methods. 2021;**18**(12):1463-1476

[5] de Jonge N, Houben L, Dunin-Borkowski RE, Ross FM. Resolution and aberration correction in liquid cell transmission electron microscopy. Nature Reviews Materials [Internet]. 2019;**4**(1):61-78. DOI: 10.1038/s41578-018-0071-2

[6] Danev R, Yanagisawa H, Kikkawa M. Cryo-electron microscopy methodology: Current aspects and future directions. Trends in Biochemical Sciences [Internet]. 2019;**44**(10):837-848. Available from:. DOI: 10.1016/j.tibs.2019.04.008

[7] Facchetti F, Bugatti M, Drera E, Tripodo C, Sartori E, Cancila V, et al. SARS-CoV2 vertical transmission with adverse effects on the newborn revealed through integrated immunohistochemical, electron microscopy and molecular analyses of Placenta. eBioMedicine. 2020;**59**:1-8

[8] Restelli F, Pollo B, Vetrano IG, Cabras S, Broggi M, Schiariti M, et al. Confocal laser microscopy in neurosurgery: State of the art of actual clinical applications. Journal of Clinical Medicine. 2021;**10**(9):1-25

[9] Slaoui M, Bauchet AL, Fiette L. Tissue sampling and processing for histopathology evaluation. Methods in Molecular Biology. 2017;**1641**:101-114

[10] Comanescu M, Annaratone L, D'Armento G, Cardos G, Sapino A, Bussolati G. Critical steps in tissue processing in histopathology. Recent Patents DNA Gene Seq. 2012;**6**(1):22-32

[11] Dewi AK, Anwar C, Komohara Y. Brain structure morphology after being fixated with ethanol on electron microscope. International Journal of Morphology. 2020;**38**(2):305-308

[12] Kiernan JA. Hassle-Free. CossMark; 1994. pp. 8-13

[13] Wittekind D. Traditional staining for routine diagnostic pathology including the role of tannic acid. 1. Value and limitations of the hematoxylin-eosin stain. Biotechnic & Histochemistry. 2003;**78**(5):261-270

[14] Dapson R, Horobin RW, Kiernan JA. Hematoxylin shortages: Their causes and duration, and other dyes that can replace hemalum in routine hematoxylin and eosin staining. Biotechnic & Histochemistry. 2010;**85**(1):55-63

[15] Ross MH, Pawlina W. Histology: A Text and Atlas with Correlated Cell and Molecular Biology. Seventh ed. Wolters Kluwer. Taylor and Francis Online; 2016

Chapter 2

Molecular Histopathology and Cytopathology in Cardiovascular Diseases

Dang Viet Duc, Nguyen Thanh Huy, Tran Quoc Quy and Nguyen Tat Tho

Abstract

In this chapter, we describe the most deadly heart diseases, including the fourth parts: Anatomy of the heart, chronic coronary syndrome and acute coronary syndrome and STEMI, Cardiomyopathy, and Pulmonary embolism. The written structure of a component includes Abstract, Pathophysiology, Clinical diagnostic criteria, histopathology, and cytopathology. The content is summarized based on the recommendations of the American Heart Association and the European Society of Cardiology. All images in this chapter are data at our center. In the chapter, we will see the relationship between histopathology and cytopathology and pathophysiology, which will serve as a basis for us to have more studies in the future.

Keywords: anatomy of the heart, coronary artery disease, cardiomyopathy, pulmonary embolism, histopathology and cytopathology

1. Introduction — Anatomy of the heart

1.1 Orientation of the heart within the thorax

The mirror image of the heart to the anterior chest wall is a quadrilateral bounded by four angles: Upper left (the second intercostal space, 1 cm from the left sternal border), upper right (the second intercostal space, 1 cm from the right sternal border), lower left (the 5th intercostal space with the left midclavicular line corresponding to the apex of the heart), and lower right (the ascending space of the rib to the right border of the sternum).

In describing the orientation of a specific organ, such as the heart, the relationships are as follows:

- Front of the heart: directly related to the sternum, the costal cartilages III-VI, the right and the left lung (**Figure 1a**).

- Diaphragm: The right atrium, right ventricle, and part of the left ventricle are directly related to the diaphragm and located in the epigastrium.

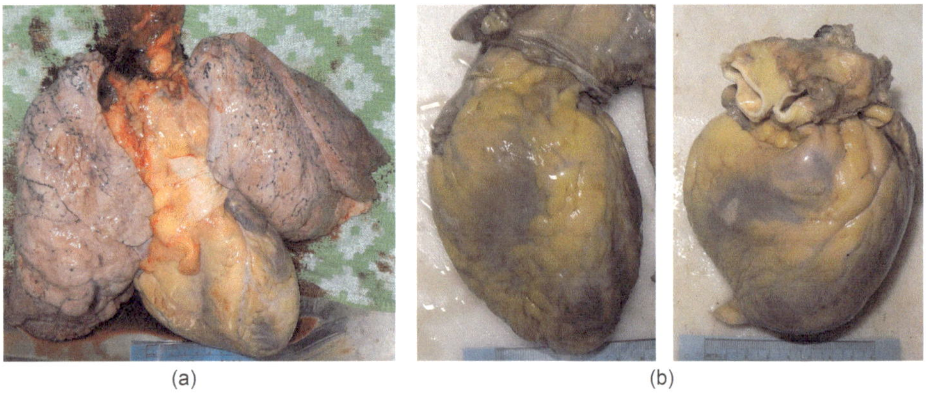

Figure 1.
(a) Heart and lung (b) Cardiac anterior view (left) and posterior view (right).

- Back of the heart: The posterior wall of the left atrium is directly related to the esophagus, so the cardiac image is clearly acquired through transesophageal echocardiography.

1.2 Major veins of the heart

- Superior vena cava: Venous return from the head, neck, and upper extremities into the right atrium through the superior vena cava.

- Inferior vena cava: from the lower abdomen to the right of the spine, this vein has a passage in the parenchyma and posterior to the liver, and receives the superior hepatic vein before into the right atrium through the inferior vena cava.

1.3 Right atrium and septum

The right atrium is directly related to the diaphragm and the substernal area below. The right atrium can be visualized as a hexadecimal volume with several notable structures and associations as follows:

- The upper surface has an orifice of the superior vena cava without the valve.

- The right atrium is shorter and more obtuse than the left atrium.

- The lower surface has the orifice of the inferior vena cava with the Eustachi valve.

- Near the orifice of the inferior vena cava, there is a coronary sinus hole, where the coronary vein drains into the right atrium from the posterior surface of the heart.

1.4 Left atrium and pulmonary veins

The left atrium is located behind and to the left of the right atrium. The left atrium and pulmonary veins are structures located in the deepest layer of the heart.

- The posterior wall of the left atrium is directly related to the esophagus posteriorly, so the intraesophageal probe can easily probe the left atrium and other anterior structures.

- The pulmonary veins (two right and two left) on both sides of the posterior wall of the left atrium. The orifice of pulmonary veins is the deepest and most difficult-to-see structure on transthoracic ultrasound.

- In the anterior wall, outside the left atrium connecting with the left atrium, is a small niche like an ear. In the left atrium, there are some ligaments. The atrium will also be enlarged when there is increased pressure in the left atrium (narrowing, mitral regurgitation...) and is the most likely place to form blood clots, especially in cases of atrial fibrillation. This thrombus may extend from the atrium into the appendage of the left atrium.

1.5 Right ventricle and Interventricular septum

The right ventricle divide structure into two parts, the first extends from the tricuspid valve is the inlet. The inlet component ejected blood to the pulmonary artery through the second part, known as the outflow portion. It is a tubular structure about 1.5 cm long with a funnel shape, the top of which is the orifice of the pulmonary valve.

The interventricular septum is a membrane and muscle that separates the two ventricles. The interventricular septum also has two parts:

- The fragile upper part (2 mm) is called the membranous portion.

- The lower part is the muscular portion (**Figure 2**).

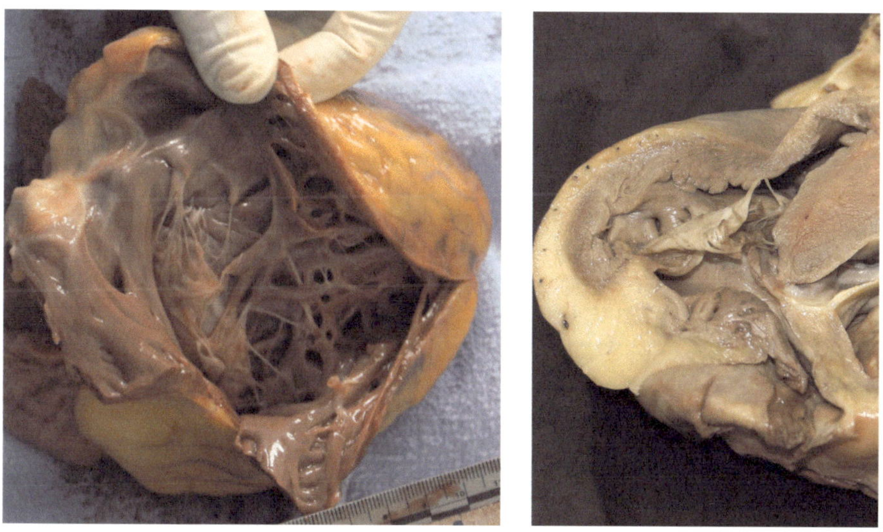

Figure 2.
Right ventricle free wall view (left) and septum view (right).

1.6 Left ventricle

The left ventricle is an essential chamber because it ejects blood into the aorta. The left ventricle is located posterior to the right ventricle, an anterior-medial part is covered by the right ventricle, separated by the interventricular septum.

- In the longitudinal view, the left ventricle has an oval shape, with the very small being the apex, the very large (bottom left ventricle) being the mitral valve and the left ventricular (LV) outflow tract.

- The LV muscle layer is much thicker than the right ventricle, on average 1 cm, and the endocardium covers the lumen.

- The LV outflow tract is the route that ejects blood from the left ventricle to the aorta, located between the interventricular septum in front and the anterior mitral leaflet posteriorly, limited from the apex of the anterior mitral valve to the aortic annulus (**Figure 3**).

1.7 Tricuspid valve

Tricuspid valve is a cardiac valve located in the right atrioventricular orifice, whose function is to open during diastole to allow blood to flow from the right atrium to the right ventricle and close during systole to prevent blood backing up into the right atrium.

- Tricuspid valve has three leaflets:

- The anterior tricuspid leaflet is the largest, and most mobile and forms an intracavitary curtain that partially separates the inflow and outflow tracts of the right ventricle.

- The posterior leaflet adheres to the posterior wall of the right ventricle.

- It is especially noticeable that the septal leaflet adheres to the interventricular septum. This leaflet attaches to the membranous portion of the septum 8–10 mm lower than the attachment of the LV mitral valve.

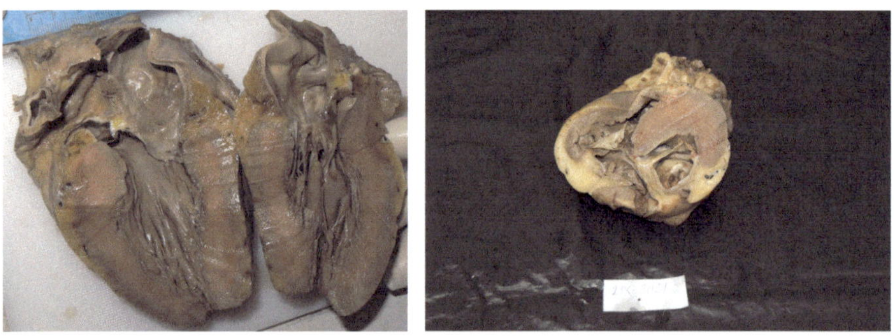

Figure 3.
Left ventricle, long axis (left), and short axis (right).

The tricuspid annulus is a fibrous ring with an average circumference of 105–120 mm. The tricuspid annulus is very often dilated when the right ventricle is dilated (as in pulmonary hypertension) causing tricuspid regurgitation.

1.8 Pulmonary valve

- Pulmonary valve is located at the orifice of the pulmonary artery and has three semicircular leaflets. These leaflets are thin fibrous membranes, two sides covered by endothelium, without ligaments like the atrioventricular valve, but only have one border attached to a fibrous ring called the pulmonary valve ring.

- Pulmonary valve ring average has approximately the circumference of the aortic valve ring from 65 to 70 mm. The size of the annulus is significant to evaluate in the tetralogy of Fallot. The pulmonary artery trunk has an oblique direction to the left shoulder, so to see the pulmonary artery trunk, when ultrasound, it is necessary to tilt the transducer slightly from the left sternal border to the left shoulder.

- The pulmonary artery trunk in regular or congenital malformations all keep anterior to posterior orientation, in contrast to the aorta, which always has an anterior direction. The division of the pulmonary artery is also known as the confluence of the right and left branches.

1.9 Mitral valve

Mitral valve is a simple name for the mitral valve apparatus, which plays an essential role in ensuring the one-way flow of blood from the left atrium to the left ventricle.

The mitral valve apparatus consists of the following components: Annulus, leaflets, subvalvular organization including chordae tendineae and papillary muscle.

- *Annulus:* This is a fibrous ring at the orifice of the mitral valve separating the left atrium and the left ventricle and is the attachment point for the leaflets. The mitral annulus has a standard elliptical shape with an anterior–posterior diameter smaller than the transverse diameter. Mitral regurgitation often leads to annular dilatation and annulus deformity because the anterior–posterior diameter is dilated more than the transverse diameter. These lesions form one of the mechanisms that cause mitral regurgitation.

- *Leaflets:* The two leaflets have a cap shape. The junction of the two leaflets near the annulus creates two valve edges, the anterolateral and posteromedial commissure. The anterior leaflet has more prominent than the posterior leaflet but has a smaller length of attachment to the ring than the attachment of the posterior leaflet. On ultrasound, identify the anterolateral commissure as which edge is closest to the lateral wall of the left ventricle and which posteromedial commissure is located near the interventricular septum.

- *Subvalvular:* The chordae tendineae are fibrous cords that radiate from the top of the papillary muscle to hold the leaflets. There are two papillary muscles arising from the inner surface of the left ventricle near the apex of the heart, the anterolateral and posteromedial papillary muscles.

1.10 Aortic valve

The aortic valve, thicker and stronger than the pulmonary valve, is composed of three components (i.e, annulus, cusps, and commissures), and consists of three leaflets named for their anatomical relationship to the coronary ostium (**Figure 4**):

- Right coronary leaflet: located anterior-right.
- Left coronary leaflet: Anterior-left.
- Non-coronary leaflet: Located posterior-right.

There is no coronary artery in the sinus of Valsalva of the Non-coronary leaflet. Three valve edges are where the three leaflets meet each other at the place of attachment to the valve ring. Valve edges may become fused in rheumatic lesions. The aortic valve ring has a circumference of 65–70 mm in adults.

1.11 Coronary arteries and veins

The right coronary artery from the sinus of Valsalva has an anterior direction in the epicardial layer and enters the right atrioventricular sulcus. The left coronary artery from the left sinus of Valsalva loops posteriorly to the pulmonary artery root, then exits anteriorly. The left main coronary artery bifurcates into the left anterior descending and left circumflex arteries. In a normal person, these arteries are usually only visible for the first 1–2 cm in the left sternal cross-section. Many cardiac veins drain into the right atrium. Most notable because ultrasound can be seen in the coronary sinus, a bulging vein that receives most of the cardiac veins before emptying into the right atrium. This sinus is about 2.5 cm long, enlarged, and located in the coronary sulcus at the back of the heart (**Figure 5**).

1.12 Pericardium

The pericardium is a conical-shaped structure that adheres to and envelops the heart, including the serous and fibrous pericardium. The fibrous pericardium is a resilient sac that surrounds the heart and attaches to the great vessels. The serous

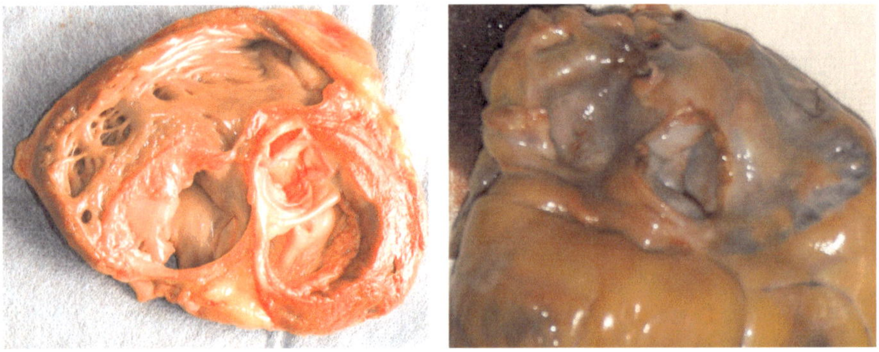

Figure 4.
Aortic valve inferior view (left) and superior view (right).

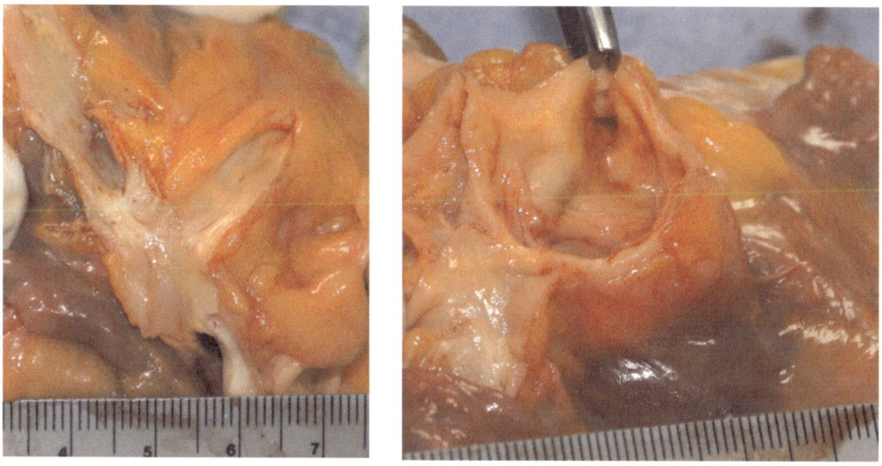

Figure 5.
The left coronary artery: left main, left anterior descending, left circumflex artery (left); ostium (right).

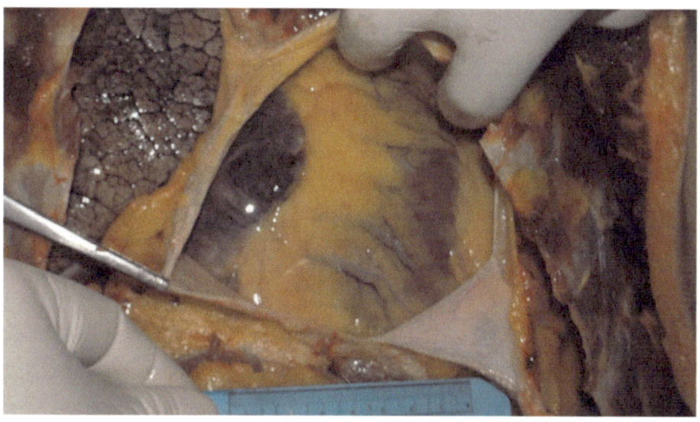

Figure 6.
Pericardium.

pericardium forms the delicate inner lining of the fibrous pericardium and continues onto the surface of the heart and great vessels at the pericardial reflection. Between the layers of the pericardium is a virtual space called the pericardial cavity. Blood and fluid can appear in this space and create a pericardial effusion (**Figure 6**).

2. Coronary artery disease

2.1 Chronic coronary syndrome

2.1.1 Abstract

Coronary artery disease (CAD) is a pathological process characterized by obstructive or non-obstructive atherosclerotic plaque accumulation in the epicardial arteries. The CAD process is dynamic and depends on the stability or instability of atherosclerotic plaques. The acute atherothrombotic event can occur at any time, caused by plaque rupture or erosion, and results in various clinical presentations, categorized as either acute coronary syndromes (ACS) or chronic coronary syndromes (CCS). The CCS is a new term accepted at the European society of cardiology congress (ESC) 2019, replacing the previous name of stable angina or stable coronary artery disease. According to ESC 2019, CCS has six clinical scenarios: (1) patients with "stable" anginal symptoms and/or dyspnea; (2) patients with newly discovered heart failure or left ventricular dysfunction; (3) patients with stabilized symptoms <1 year after an ACS, or patients with recent revascularization; (4) more than one year after initial diagnosis or revascularization; (5) patients with angina and suspected vasospastic or microvascular disease; (6) CAD is detected at screening without any symptom [1].

2.1.2 Pathophysiology

CCS is a condition involving the relative stability of coronary atherosclerotic plaques, in the absence of an acute atherothrombotic event caused by plaque rupture or erosion. When progressive atherosclerotic plaques cause significant narrowing of the lumen of the coronary arteries (usually above 70% of the lumen diameter), symptoms can be present, most typically angina/shortness of breath during physical exertion and relief at rest [2].

When the lumen of a coronary artery is narrowed, the myocardial perfusion by this vessel is significantly reduced. Especially during physical exertion, the oxygen supply to the heart muscle is impaired while the oxygen demand increases. With this supply–demand imbalance, the heart muscle must depend on anaerobic metabolism to ensure normal function. It is anaerobic metabolic products such as LDH and adenosine that cause chest pain by stimulating the nerve endings of the coronary system. The long-term consequences of this ischemic heart condition are angina attacks during physical exertion, seriously affecting the quality of life as well as the patient's psyche; it may cause impaired LV function and risk of arrhythmias [3]. In addition to the main cause of myocardial hypoxia due to atherosclerosis which causes the narrowing of the coronary vessels, other factors such as vasospasm, especially small blood vessels, anemia, and decreased blood oxygen are also important causes of angina [4]. Factors affecting myocardial oxygen demand are heart rate, myocardial contractility, preload, and afterload. The increase in these factors increases the oxygen demand of the heart muscle and affects myocardial ischemia. Therefore, for the treatment of CCS, increased supply and/or decrease in myocardial oxygen demand along with antiplatelet therapy are core issues [1].

2.1.3 Clinical diagnostic criteria

Angina pectoris: In the diagnosis of CAD, angina is the most important clinical symptom to help with diagnosis, although chest pain has many different causes, so it is necessary to distinguish whether chest pain is caused by coronary heart disease or not. Typical chest pain includes the following characteristics:

- Location: usually behind the sternum and as an area rather than a point, pain can spread to the neck, shoulders, hands, epigastric, or back. Commonly it spreads to the left shoulder or hand.

- Circumstances of appearance: when exerting, having strong emotions, experiencing cold, after a lavish meal, or smoking. Some cases of angina may occur at night, when changing positions, or with tachycardia.

- Character: The pain is like tightening, strangulation, or being weighed down in front of the chest. It may be accompanied by a feeling of shortness of breath, headache, nausea, or sweating. The pain usually lasts about a few minutes (3–5 minutes), it can be longer but usually no more than 20 minutes (when you need to think about acute coronary syndrome). Pains that last less than 1 minute should be caused by another reason rather than the heart [5].

- Investigations such as electrocardiogram, echocardiography, and hs-troponin tests help to rule out acute coronary syndrome as well as other causes of chest pain such as aortic valve stenosis, obstructive hypertrophic cardiomyopathy, aortic dissection… [1, 6].

2.1.4 Histopathology

The most common cause of CCS is atherosclerotic coronary artery obstruction. The microscopic grading of atherosclerosis can be classified according to the Modified American Heart Association criteria [7].

- Pathological intimal thickening: characterized by acellular lipid pools within the intima. No lipid core.

- Fibrous cap atheroma: a lipid core containing extracellular lipid cholesterol crystals and necrotic debris covered by a thick, sometimes multilayered, cap of fibrous tissue. Punctate or patchy calcification. Lymphocytic infiltration may be prominent, especially at the edge of cores.

- Thin fibrous cap atheroma: a thin, occasionally inflamed, fibrous cap covers a lipid core. <65 μm in thickness in the coronary, <200 μm in the carotid arteries. The thin fibrous cap atheroma is a plaque that is considered unstable, with a high risk of rupture, and is also known as "vulnerable plaque".

- Plaque rupture: clear evidence of ruptured fibrous cap and luminal thrombus formation which communicates with the underlying necrotic core.

- Plaque erosion: a fibrous cap atheroma with luminal thrombus as above, but the thrombus formation overly area lacking surface endothelium. Erosion may be seen in early lesions, such as pathological intimal thickening.

- Fibrocalcific lesion: "stable" lesion, a dense collagen plaque containing a large area of calcification and a few scattered smooth muscle cells. This is a consequence of the dystrophic calcification of the lipid core.

- Calcified nodule: heavily calcified lesion, probably one of the last stages of the atherosclerotic process.

- Coronary atheromas may have a focal appearance. The irregular plaques vary both in size and stenosis from place to place, and are often eccentric, resulting in a segmented crescent-shaped lumen artery (**Figures** 7 and 8).

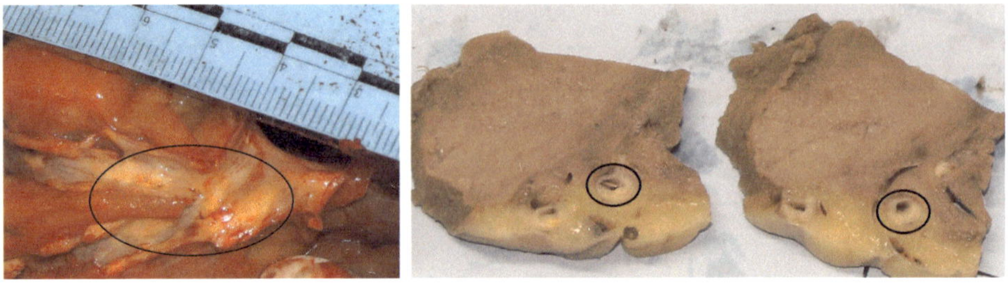

Figure 7.
Histopathology of CCS.

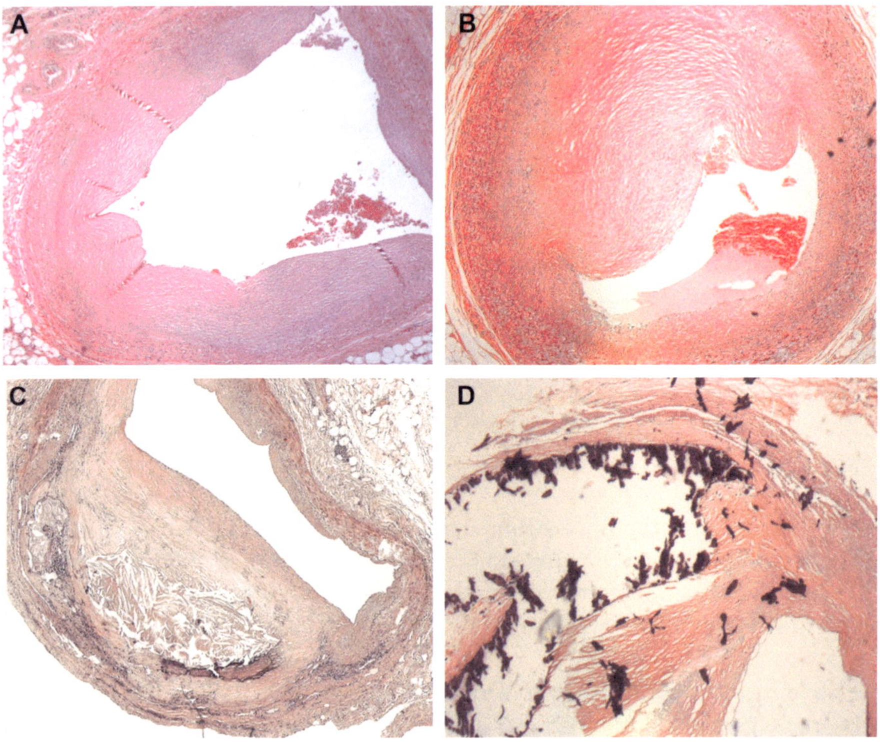

Figure 8.
Micrographs showing the coronary tree. A, the fat tissue in the adventitia (H&E, 100X). B, the severe narrowing lumen by atherosclerotic plaque, with several hemorrhagic necrotic cores and deposition of lipids and infiltration of lipid-laden foam cells in the tunica intima and tunica media (H&E, 100X). C, Panel indicates histological findings features of fibrous cap atheroma with fibrous tissue, necrotic core, and calcification (H&E, 100X). D, intraplaque hemorrhage with the necrotic core with a form of calcification that results in irregular nodules of calcium (H&E, 100X).

2.2 Non-ST elevation acute coronary syndrome

2.2.1 Abstract

Non-ST elevation acute coronary syndrome consists of two clinical scenarios: non-ST elevation myocardial infarction (NSTEMI) and unstable angina. Clinically and in the electrocardiogram, there is no difference between them, the distinction is in NSTEMI, there is an increase in myocardial biomarkers. The treatment of NSTEMI differs fundamentally from ST-elevation myocardial infarction in approach strategy, time of intervention, and treatment modalities with or without fibrinolysis. An acute coronary syndrome is a severe event of CAD that is the leading cause of cardiovascular death and morbidity. In particular, NSTEMI still accounts for the leading proportion of acute coronary events in developed countries and worldwide. There have been many advances in the effective diagnosis and treatment of acute coronary artery syndrome. However, this is still a severe disease and needs attention [8].

2.2.2 Pathophysiology

The mechanism of ACS is due to the instability of the atherosclerotic plaque and the plaque rupture or erosion. If a large rupture and massive blood clot formation fill the entire lumen of the vessel, it will lead to a transmural myocardial infarction or STEMI. If the rupture is smaller and the clot has not yet led to a complete blockage of a coronary artery, it is unstable angina and NSTEMI. In addition, the mechanisms of the movement of small thrombosis to cause occlusion of microvascular and contraction further aggravate myocardial ischemia. The formation of blood clots occurs due to a cracked atherosclerotic plaque that reveals the subendothelial matrix, which activates the GP IIb/IIIa receptors on the platelet surface when it comes into contact with platelets, causing platelets to aggregate, thereby initiating a blood clotting cascade [9].

The consequence of the above phenomena is a serious and rapid decrease in blood flow to the myocardial area perfused by that coronary artery, clinically manifested as unstable angina pectoris, on the electrocardiogram is an image of acute myocardial ischemia with ST depression or sharp, negative T wave, elevated cardiac enzymes (troponin, CK-MB) [10–12].

2.2.3 Clinical diagnostic criteria

- Clinical: Symptoms of coronary chest pain are the same as in stable angina, although there are differences in the nature of the pain: unstable angina is usually more intense, lasts longer (more than 20 minutes), pain may occur during rest, with no or little response to nitrate [8].

- Electrocardiogram: During the pain, changes in the ST segment can be seen, most commonly ST depression, negative or reversal T wave. Up to 20% of patients do not have immediate changes on the electrocardiogram, so it is recommended to have ECG repeatedly [10].

- Myocardial biomarker: in MI, there is often an increase in hs Troponin I or T, CK, CK-MB [12, 13].

- Echocardiography: helps evaluate regional dyskinesia, LV function, and accompanying heart valve diseases [14].

2.3 Acute ST-elevation myocardial infarction

2.3.1 Abstract

Acute myocardial infarction (MI) is one of the leading causes of death in the US and European countries. It is estimated that in the US every year about 1 million patients are hospitalized and 200,000–300,000 deaths from acute MI. In recent years, advances in diagnosis and treatment have significantly reduced mortality from acute MI. The introduction of the coronary care unit (CCU) in the early 60s, followed by thrombolytic drugs in the 80s, and now percutaneous coronary interventions with advances in drugs therapy has reduced the mortality rate worldwide from about >30% in the past to <7% in the 2000s [15].

2.3.2 Pathophysiology

MI is caused by a complete blockage of one or more coronary artery branches causing sudden myocardial ischemia and necrosis of the myocardial area perfused by that branch of the coronary artery. The main mechanism that causes this phenomenon is the instability and rupture or erosion of the atherosclerotic plaque that causes the formation of thrombosis that fills the entire lumen of the vessels, which abruptly stops the flow of blood to nourish the myocardial area behind that and quickly leads to necrosis [9]. This necrotic process can be rapid or slow depending on whether the patient has previous collateral circulation or not [16]. More than 50% of acute MI occur on previous atherosclerotic lesions that cause only mild stenosis [17]. If the rupture causes the formation of a blood clot that is not large, and has not yet filled the entire lumen of the vessels, then the clinical manifestation is unstable angina. MI is also expanded when there is necrosis of the myocardial area associated with hypoperfusion due to other causes such as acute blood loss and severe hypotension in septic shock (**Figure 9**).

2.3.3 Clinical diagnostic criteria

The definition of myocardial infarction denotes the presence of acute myocardial injury detected by abnormal cardiac biomarkers in the setting of evidence of acute myocardial ischemia. Diagnostic criteria for MI include an increase or decrease of myocardial biomarker (specifically cardiac troponin) and one of the following conditions:

- Symptoms of acute myocardial ischemia include chest pain, shortness of breath...
- New electrocardiographic transformations associated with myocardial ischemia such as ST elevation, ST depression, and pathological Q waves.
- Images of new regional wall motion abnormality on ultrasound, CMR.
- Identification of a coronary thrombus by angiography or autopsy (**Figure 10**) [18].

2.4 Histopathology and cytopathology of myocardial infarction

Early in an infarct (1–3 hours), myocytes may have a wavy appearance, and there may be interstitial edema (**Figure 11A**). Increased eosinophilic staining of myocytes is

DOI: http://dx.doi.org/10.5772/intechopen.110503

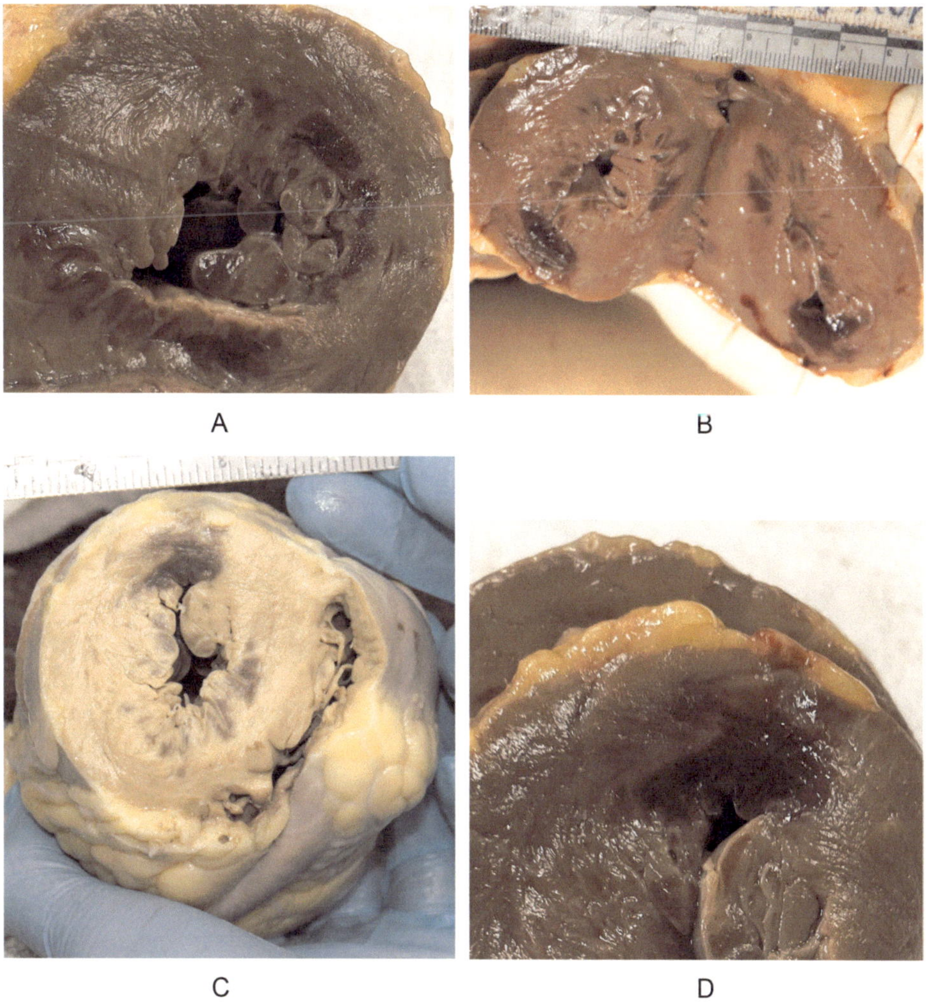

Figure 9.
A regional or focal MI.

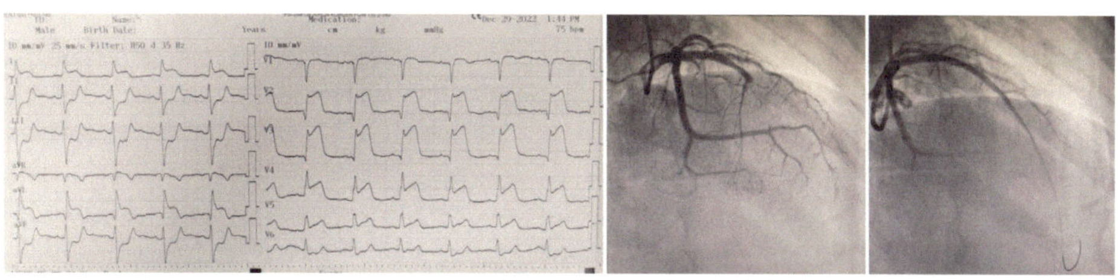

Figure 10.
ECG anterior STEMI (left); coronary thrombus and percutaneous coronary intervention of left anterior descending (right).

usually accompanied by contraction band necrosis and loss of myocyte nuclei (**Figure 11B**). These histologic changes can be appreciated by 4–12 hours, then infiltrated by inflammatory cells. Early ischemia, defined as the first 72 hours, is

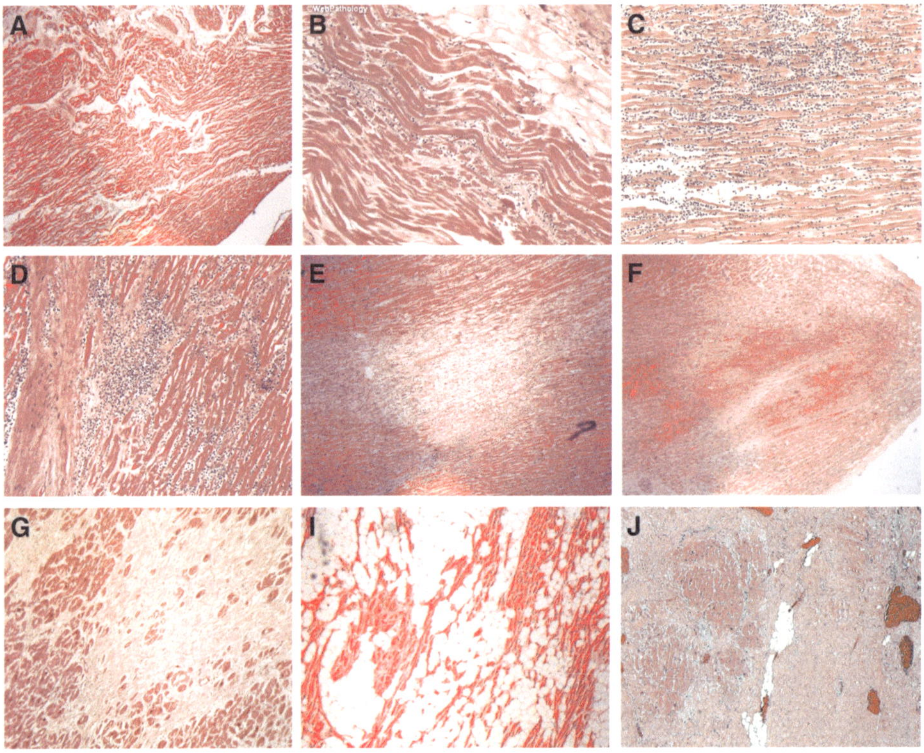

Figure 11.
Histopathology of myocardial infarction.

hallmarked by the first arrival of neutrophils as they marginate through the blood vessels and can be seen in perivascular spaces. Within the first 24–48 hours, neutrophils increase within the interstitium (**Figure 11C**); these interstitial neutrophils mainly stay intact during the first 48 hours. And within 48–72 hours, the degeneration of neutrophils begins. In other words, there is an approximately equal mix of intact and degenerating neutrophils within the first 24–72 hours of early ischemia. When it is closer to 72 hours, degenerating neutrophils and abundant cellular debris start to predominate (**Figure 11D**).

Around the third day (72 hours), there is early removal of myocytes, and the interstitial cells consist of lymphocytes, pigment-laden histiocytes, and myofibroblasts. There has been no appearance of collagen. Over the next stage of five to seven days, interstitial cells continue to proliferate. This is the most cellular stage of the healing process with a large number of interstitial inflammatory cells (**Figure 11E** and **F**). After about two to four weeks, inflammatory cells begin to decrease gradually, and collagen deposition increases (**Figure 11G**). After one to two months, only a few inflammatory cells remain, and collagen is firmly established (**Figure 11H**). After a period of two months, the inflammation ceases, and there is only a dense layer of collagen; the scar is formed. Basically, an infarct does not progress further after two months, although a well-healed scar may undergo additional changes, such as fatty infiltration and neovascularization. However, these are more variable features. There are usually remaining myocytes entrapped within areas of a healed infarct's scar, and this is a potential focus of arrhythmias (**Figure 11I** and **J**).

DOI: http://dx.doi.org/10.5772/intechopen.110503

3. Cardiomyopathy

Cardiomyopathy is a group of structural disorders of the myocardium. Unlike other structural heart disorders such as coronary artery disease, valvular heart disease, and congenital heart disease. Cardiomyopathy is classified into three main types based on pathological features.

3.1 Dilated cardiomyopathy

3.1.1 Abstract

Dilated cardiomyopathy is a myocardial dysfunction causing heart failure in which ventricular dilatation and systolic dysfunction predominate. Symptoms include dyspnea, fatigue, and peripheral edema. Diagnosis is based on clinical findings, quantification of natriuretic peptide (BNP) levels, chest x-ray, echocardiography, and CMR. Treatment of dilated cardiomyopathy is based on etiology. If heart failure is advanced and severe, cardiac resynchronization therapy (CRT), implantable cardioverter defibrillator (ICD), moderate to severe regurgitation repair, LV assist device may be needed in the short-term or long-term and heart transplant [19]. Dilated cardiomyopathy can develop at any age but is more common in adults under age 50. In the United States, men are three times more likely to have the disease than women, and African-Americans are three times more likely to have the disease than whites; about 5 to 8 out of 100,000 people get it each year [20].

3.1.2 Pathophysiology

As primary cardiomyopathy, dilated cardiomyopathy has been identified in the absence of other disorders that can cause dilated cardiomyopathy, malformations such as severe coronary artery disease or hypertension, or valvular heart disease. In some patients, dilated cardiomyopathy is thought to progress from acute myocarditis (often viral etiology in most cases), followed by a latent phase, a stage of disseminated cell death, cardiomyocytes (causing an autoimmune response to virally altered cardiomyocytes), and fibrosis. Regardless of the cause, the myocardium dilates, enlarges, and enlarges to compensate [19, 21]. The disorder affects both the left and right ventricles in most patients but rarely affects only one ventricle. Thrombosis can form due to blood stagnation when time dilates and cardiac dysfunction is significant.

3.1.3 Clinical diagnostic criteria

Diagnosis of dilated cardiomyopathy is based on history, physical examination, and exclusion of other common causes of ventricular dysfunction (eg, hypertension, primary valvular disease, coronary artery disease) by the chest x-ray, electrocardiogram, echocardiography, and cardiac magnetic resonance imaging (CMR). Endocardial biopsies are performed in some cases. In cases of unknown etiology, family members are screened for cardiac dysfunction to detect early-onset heart disease, heart failure, or sudden death (such as echocardiography).

- Serological tests for Toxoplasma, Trigonoscuta cruzi, coxsackievirus, HIV, and echovirus may be performed in appropriate cases.

- Chest X-ray showed an enlarged heart. Pleural effusion, most commonly on the right side, is often associated with pulmonary hypertension and interstitial edema.

- The electrocardiogram usually shows sinus tachycardia and nonspecific ST-segment depression with low voltage or T wave inversion. Occasionally, pathological Q waves appear in the precordial leads, indicating a previous myocardial infarction. Left bundle branch block and atrial fibrillation are common.

- Echocardiography helps to rule out primary valvular disease and shows left ventricular dilation and systolic dysfunction with impaired global contractility or right ventricular dysfunction or functional mitral and tricuspid regurgitation. Echocardiography may also show chamber thrombosis.

- CMR is useful in providing detailed images of myocardial structure and function. CMR with gadolinium contrast agent may show structural abnormalities of the myocardium or scar tissue. CMR can help diagnose active myocarditis, sarcoidosis, muscular dystrophy, or Chagas disease). Positron emission tomography (PET) is highly sensitive for the diagnosis of sarcoidosis.

- Coronary angiography to rule out coronary artery disease. Patients with angina or with certain cardiovascular risk factors and elderly patients are more likely to develop coronary artery disease. Endomyocardial biopsy is indicated if giant cell myocarditis, eosinophilic myocarditis, or sarcoidosis are suspected, as the results will influence the treatment [19, 22].

3.1.4 Histopathology and cytopathology

Dilated cardiomyopathy is a progressive, diffuse process involving cardiomyocytes from the right and left ventricles, resulting in both chambers becoming dilated and dysfunctional. As the myocardium relaxes, it becomes stretchy and thinner. Consequently, the ventricular chamber widens. Since this condition's histologic features are nonspecific, it is a microscopic diagnosis of exclusion. Previous studies have also established such findings, but only in the myocardium of patients with end-stage disease (**Figure 12**).

- Microscopic description: Myocytes have normal architectural distribution but changes in numbers, sizes, and shapes, as well as in the cytoplasm and nucleus. With regards to the size of myocytes, there are significant large variations, as these are a combination of hypertrophic, atrophic, and normal myocardiocytes or are associated with degenerative changes. Due to the atrophy of the myocytes, they have an appearance of long and thin fibers, with a sinuous path and a characteristic appearance of "corrugated fibers" (**Figure 13A**). These fibers are separated from each other by loose spaces, a suggestive aspect of edematous infiltration of the interstitia. The typical atrophy is presented with zonal characters, rarely with extensive or focal elements.

Fibrosis is diffuse or focal in the interstitial or perivascular topography. In interstitia, the fibrillar collagen's presence in intermuscular spaces normally devoid of collagen is noticed. The distribution pattern can vary from a fine peri-myocyte distribution to massive scars. In the case of perivascular fibrosis, collagen has

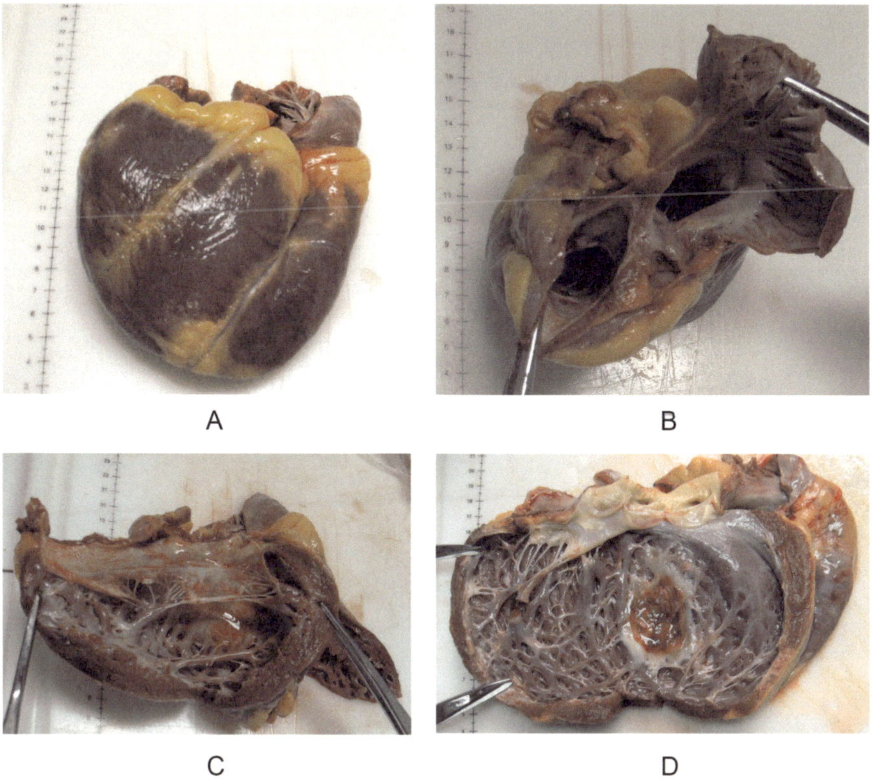

Figure 12.
Dilated cardiomyopathy.

accumulated in the adventitia of intramedullary coronary arteries and arterioles, otherwise remains untouched (**Figure 13B**). The presence of fatty tissue infiltrates (lipomatosis) with focal characters. (**Figure 13C**). Collagen has individually surrounded the myocardial fibers with a "ragged" appearance due to the corrugated cell membrane (**Figure 13D**).

3.2 Hypertrophic cardiomyopathy

3.2.1 Abstract

Hypertrophic cardiomyopathy (HCM) is a congenital or acquired disorder characterized by marked ventricular hypertrophy and diastolic dysfunction but no increased afterload. Symptoms include difficulty breathing, chest pain, fainting, and even sudden death. HCM is diagnosed based on echocardiography and CMR. The initial therapy is beta-blockers, verapamil, disopyramide, alcohol septal ablation, or surgical removal of outlet obstruction [23].

3.2.2 Pathophysiology

Cardiac muscle abnormalities with fibrous tissue and not specific to HCM. The most common is marked hypertrophy and thickening of the anterior septum and the adjacent

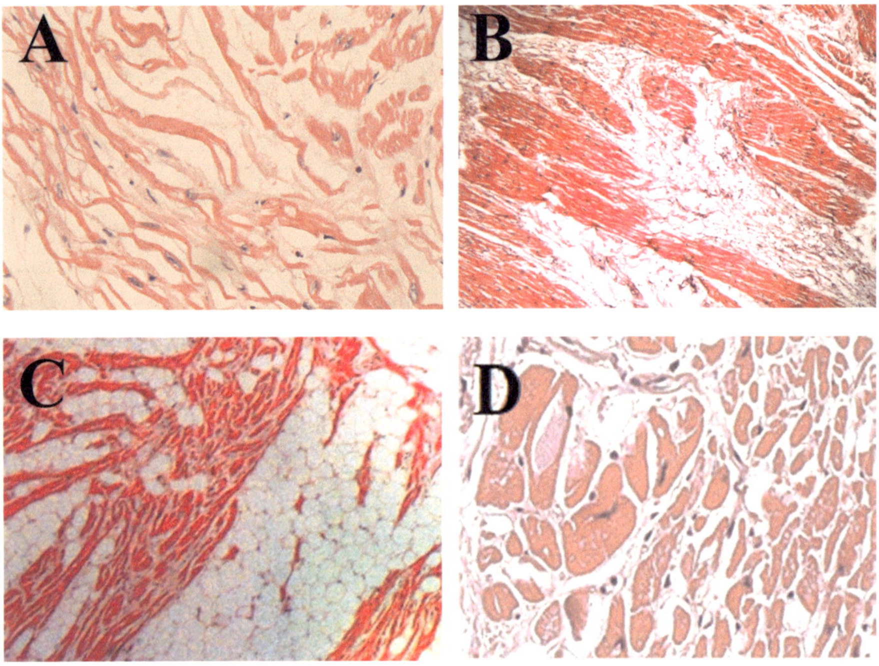

Figure 13.
Microscopic diagnosis dilated cardiomyopathy.

anterior free wall below the aortic valve, with little or no LV posterior wall hypertrophy. Occasionally, isolated apical hypertrophy occurs; most cases are asymmetric hypertrophy, and a few cases of symmetrical hypertrophy have been reported [24].

Two-thirds of patients present with "congestion" at rest or with exercise; obstruction results from mechanical resistance to the LV outflow tract during systole due to the mitral valve's forward motion (SAM). During this period, the mitral valve and valvular structures are drawn into the LV outflow tract due to the Venturi effect of high-velocity blood flow, resulting in flow obstruction and decreased cardiac output. Mitral regurgitation can also occur due to the deformed movement of the leaflets. This blockage and regurgitation cause symptoms associated with heart failure. Less commonly, left midventricular hyperplasia causes elevation of pressure gradient at the site of the papillary muscles [23, 25].

Initially, contractility is completely normal, resulting in a normal ejection fraction (EF). Thereafter, EF increases because the ventricular volume is small and empties almost completely to maintain cardiac output. Hypertrophy leads to a rigid, elastic ventricular chamber that interferes with diastolic filling, increasing end-diastolic pressure and increasing pulmonary venous pressure. As filling resistance and cardiac output decrease, the condition is worsened by any output gradient. Tachycardia allows less time to fill, so symptoms tend to appear mainly with exercise or a rapid heart rate.

Coronary blood flow may be impaired, causing angina, syncope, or arrhythmia in the absence of epicardial coronary artery injury. Impaired flow due to inadequate capillary versus muscle cell density (capillary/muscle imbalance) or narrowing of the lumen of the coronary arteries in the myocardium due to hyperplasia and hypertrophy endothelium and mesothelium. A mismatch between supply and demand can also arise due to increased oxygen demand, hypertrophy, and adverse loading conditions [23]. In some situations, myocytes die due to ischemia, will be replaced by diffuse fibrosis. Subsequently, the ventricles become enlarged with pre-existing diastolic dysfunction and progressive systolic dysfunction.

3.2.3 Clinical diagnostic criteria

The diagnosis of HCM is suspected based on murmurs and other typical symptoms, especially if the patient has unexplained syncope or a family history of sudden death. HCM must be differentiated from aortic stenosis and coronary artery disease because they have similar clinical symptoms.

- Electrocardiograms in patients with HCM often show LV hypertrophy. Abnormal Q waves in leads I, aVL, V5, and V6 are often present with asymmetrical septal hypertrophy; QRS complexes in V1 and V2, similar to previous septal infarction. Inverted, symmetrical, and deep T waves with ST-segment depression in leads DI, aVL, V5, and V6. P waves are usually broad and notched in leads DII, III, and aVF, with biphasic P waves in leads V1 and V2, indicating left atrial hypertrophy; Bundle branch block is common [26].

- Two-dimensional Doppler echocardiography and CMR help to differentiate other forms of cardiomyopathy and predict the severity of hypertrophy and LV outflow tract obstruction. It also helps to monitor the effectiveness of treatment or surgery. Exercise testing and 24-hour ambulatory ECG outpatient follow-up are recommended during the initial evaluation and every 1 to 2 years to evaluate the risk of sudden cardiac death and guide arrhythmia treatment.

- Cardiac catheterization is usually performed when invasive treatment is considered. Usually, the patient has concomitant coronary artery disease.

- Genetic markers do not affect the treatment or identification of high-risk individuals. However, genetic testing helps screen family members.

3.2.4 Histopathology

Myocyte hypertrophy is correlated with heart size. The disarray of the overall architecture of the hypertrophied myocytes characterizes histopathology in patients with HCM. It notes that whether myocytes may be obviously or barely noticeably enlarged depends on their relative heart size.

The increase in myocytes and interstitial tissue leads to increased myocardial mass. Meanwhile, the heart may or may not increase in overall size due to the hypertrophy of myocytes may or may not be associated with dilation. Dilation is a prominent feature in response to volume overload rather than pressure overload. Regarding pressure overload, the walls may be thick with no dilation, and the chamber volume ratio to wall thickness decreases; this is also known as “concentric hypertrophy”. Although the ventricular wall thickness is measured as a reflection of the degree of hypertrophy, such measurement does not accurately reflect the myocardial mass in hypertrophy with dilation (**Figure 14**).

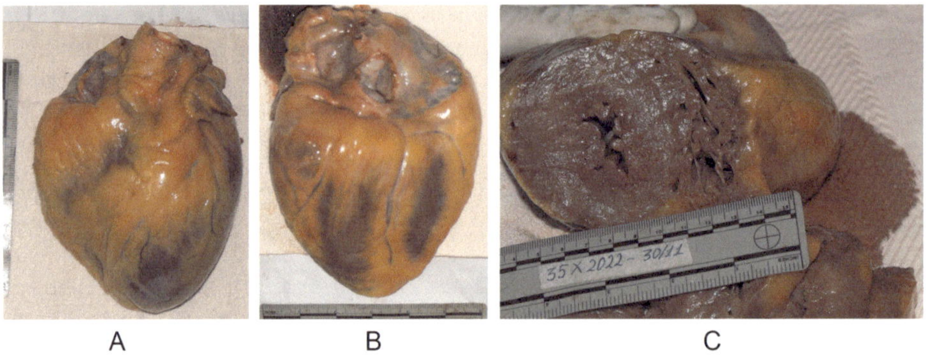

Figure 14.
Very large heart size (18 x 15 cm). Cross section of hypertrophic heart in an adult: The right ventricular free wall thickness is 1,5 cm, the LV is 3,5 cm, and the septum 3 cm.

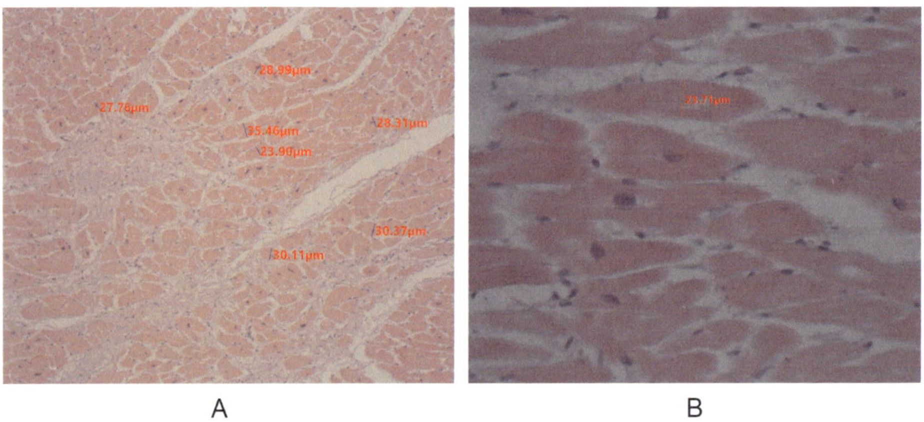

Figure 15.
In Myocardial hypertrophy cardiocyte diameter is up to 25 μm and in severe hypertrophy is usually between 25 and 30 μm.

The diameter of the myocardial cell is also an indicator that predicts different levels of hypertrophy. Under normal conditions, the myocardial cell ranges from 5 to 12 μm in diameter. In cases of mild and moderate hypertrophy, it can go up to 20 μm and 25 μm, respectively. Diameters between 25 and 30 μm usually indicate moderate to severe hypertrophy. And when diameters are greater than 30 μm, severe hypertrophy must be suspected. HCM almost always presents with cell hypertrophy. Hypertrophic myocardial cells show nuclear enlargement, bizarre nuclei, and binucleation (**Figure 15**).

The typical histologic description of hyperchromatic nuclei is like a rectangular shape, or "box-car" nuclei (**Figure 16A**). Myocardial fibrosis can be comprised of three main categories: interstitial, perivascular, and replacement-type fibrosis. In interstitial diffuse fibrosis, bundles of collagen surround the cardiomyocytes individually (**Figure 16B**). Perivascular fibrosis spreads radially around capillary and small arteries. Replacement by adipose tissue is often seen in the terminal stage of fibrosis (**Figure 16C**). Replacement fibrosis is characterized as areas of fibrosis not large enough to be considered an infarct, typically less than 3 mm in size (**Figure 16D**).

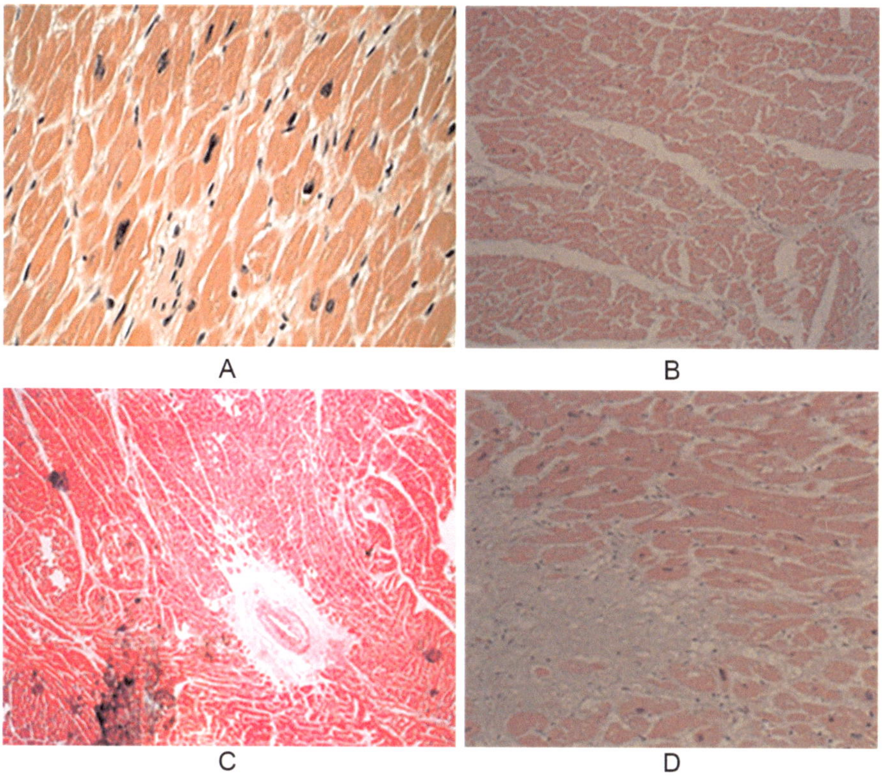

Figure 16.
A: Hyperchromatic nuclei. B: interstitial fibrosis. C: Perivascular fibrosis. D: Replacement fibrosis.

3.3 Restrictive cardiomyopathy

3.3.1 Abstract

Restrictive cardiomyopathy is the least common form of cardiomyopathy. It is characterized by noncompliant ventricular walls that resist diastolic filling; the right or left ventricle or both may be affected. Symptoms include fatigue and shortness of breath, especially with exertion. Restrictive cardiomyopathy is diagnosed based on echocardiography and cardiac catheterization. The medication is often less effective. Surgery is sometimes beneficial [27]. It classifies as non-obstructive (infiltration of the myocardium by an abnormal substance) and fibrosis (fibrosis of the endocardium and subendocardium).

3.3.2 Pathophysiology

Endocardial thickening or myocardial infiltration (with possible myocardial cell death, papillary infiltration, myocardial hypertrophy, and fibrosis) occurs on one side, typically the left or both ventricles. Thus, causing mitral or tricuspid regurgitation. If the nodal and conduction tissues are affected, the sinus node and the atrioventricular node become less functional, sometimes causing varying degrees of SA and AV block. The hemodynamic consequences are diastolic dysfunction with ventricular stiffness, loss of elasticity, impaired diastolic filling capacity, and increased filling pressure, leading to increased pulmonary venous pressure. The systolic function may worsen. A cardiac chamber thrombus can form, leading to systemic embolism [27].

3.3.3 Clinical diagnostic criteria

Restrictive cardiomyopathy should be suspected in patients with heart failure and preserved ejection fraction, particularly in the presence of systemic disease. An electrocardiogram, chest x-ray, and routine echocardiography are required.

ECG presentation is less specific and may show ST segment and T wave abnormalities and sometimes low voltage. Pathological Q wave, not due to previous myocardial infarction. LV hypertrophy due to compensatory myocardial hypertrophy or both atrioventricular block, and sinoatrial block may be present.

On a chest X-ray, the heart is usually normal in size but may be enlarged in amyloidosis or hemochromatosis. Echocardiography showed a normal LV ejection fraction. Tissue Doppler imaging often shows increased LV filling pressure, and longitudinal decline in contractile function despite normal ejection fraction. In addition, other nonspecific signs such as atrial dilatation and myocardial hypertrophy. In amyloidosis, abnormal echogenic tissue can be observed from the myocardium, and identification of the amyloid type has implications for treatment, genetic counseling, and prognosis [27, 28].

3.4 Some other diseases

In addition to the three common types mentioned above, there may also be other forms such as arrhythmogenic right ventricular cardiomyopathy, Takotsubo cardiomyopathy, peripartum cardiomyopathy, spongiform cardiomyopathy, or secondary cardiomyopathies. Consequences of endocrine, metabolic, neurological, nutritional, autoimmune, toxicological diseases... For each of these diseases, there are separate pathophysiological mechanisms and different diagnostic procedures. Histopathology is diverse, but all have in common that is, leading to cardiovascular mortality or severe cardiac dysfunction.

4. Pulmonary embolism

4.1 Abstract

Pulmonary embolism is caused by the thrombus moving through, most commonly from the large veins of the lower extremities or pelvis. Risk factors for PE are venous stasis, endothelial damage, and disorders associated with hypercoagulability [29]. Symptoms of PE include dyspnea, chest pain, and in more severe cases syncope, respiratory failure, and cardiac arrest. Physical examination may tachypnea, tachycardia, and, in more severe cases, hypotension. Computed tomographic pulmonary angiography is considered the gold standard diagnostic modality for PE with a sensitivity of 83% and specificity of 96%, although ventilation/perfusion is sometimes required. Treatment of PE with anticoagulants and thrombolytics is systemic or directly through the catheter, thrombectomy with mechanical and surgical instruments. When anticoagulation is contraindicated, an inferior vena cava filter should be placed. Preventive measures include anticoagulation and/or the use of compression stockings and lower extremity decompression devices [30].

4.2 Pathophysiology

As deep vein thrombosis develops, the clots can move through the venous system to the right heart and the pulmonary arteries, where they partially or completely obstruct one or more arterial branches of the pulmonary vessels. The severity depends on the size and amount of the thrombosis, the underlying lung condition, right ventricular function, and the fibrinolytic system's ability to dissolve the clot. The death occurred due to right ventricular failure [29, 30].

Small emboli may have no physiological effects, dissolve immediately, and resolve spontaneously within hours or days. Larger emboli can cause reflex hyperventilation, hypoxia due to inadequate ventilation/perfusion (V/Q), and low venous mixed oxygen due to decreased cardiac output. Low blood pressure, atelectasis due to decreased alveolar CO and surfactant abnormalities, and increased pulmonary vascular resistance due to mechanical obstruction and vasoconstriction lead to tachycardia and hypotension. Endogenous lysis reduces most thrombi, even moderate-sized ones, and physiological changes subside after hours or days. Some emboli are resistant to lysis and can organize and persist, subsequently causing chronic pulmonary hypertension [31, 32]. PE can be classified according to risk:

- High-risk (super-massive): Impaired RV function with hypotension/ severe respiratory failure requiring treatment with vasopressors and high-flow oxygen.

- High risk (massive): Decreased RV function causing hypotension, as defined by systolic blood pressure < 90 mm Hg or decrease in systolic blood pressure 40 mm Hg from baseline over 15 minutes.

- Intermediate risk (submasive): Decreased RV function and/or elevated troponin and/or natriuretic peptide (BNP) levels without hypotension. The European Society of Cardiology defines intermediate-risk PE as patients with a simplified PE severity index (sPESI) > 0.

- Low risk: No RV failure and no hypotension (and according to the European Society of Cardiology, sPESI score = 0) [33].

In 1 to 4% of cases, chronic residual obstruction leads to pulmonary hypertension. This condition can progress and lead to chronic right-sided heart failure [34]. When a large embolus blocks the major pulmonary arteries, or many smaller emboli combine to occlude >50% of the more distal vessels, RV pressure increases, induce in acute RV failure. The risk of death depends on the degree and rate of elevation of RV pressure and the patient's baseline cardiopulmonary status. Patients with pre-existing cardiopulmonary disease are at increased risk of mortality, but young and/or otherwise healthy patients may survive after thrombosis occluding >50% of the pulmonary vascular bed [30, 35].

Pulmonary infarction (ischemia of lung tissue) occurs in <10% of patients with a diagnosis of PE. This low incidence is attributed to the dual blood supply to the lungs (i.e, bronchi and lungs). In general, pulmonary infarctions are caused by emboli. Smaller occlusions lodge in the more distant pulmonary arteries and are almost completely reversible; pulmonary infarction is detected early by highly sensitive radiographic criteria, often before necrosis occurs.

4.3 Clinical diagnostic criteria

The clinical presentation of PE is nonspecific, which, like many other conditions, makes diagnosis more difficult. Therefore, the current diagnostic method is to assess the risk of PE, thereby recommending appropriate follow-up tests to confirm the diagnosis. According to Ceriani et al., there is currently no best model, although many probabilistic models have been developed to help clinicians easily access the diagnosis of PE. It is recommended to use a scale that is widely used in studies (such as the Wells and Geneva criteria) (**Table 1**) [31].

Wells score		**Revised Geneva score**	
Variable	**Points**	**Variable**	**Points**
Predisposing factors		Predisposing factors	
Previous DVT or PE	+1.5	Age >65	+1
Recent surgery/ immobilization	+1.5	Previous DVT or PE	+3
Cancer	+1	Surgery or fracture Within 1 month	+2
		Active malignancy	+2
Symptoms		Symptoms	
Haemoptysis	+1	Unilateral lower limb pain	+3
		Haemoptysis	+2
Clinical signs		Clinical signs	
Heart rate >100/min	+1.5	Heart rate	+3
		75–94/min	+5
		≥ 95/min	+5
Clinical signs of DVT	+3		
Clinical judgement			
Alternative diagnosis less than PE	+3	Pain can lower limb deep vein at palpation and unilateral oedema	+4
Clinical probability	Total	Clinical probability	Total
Low	0–1	Low	0–3
Intermediate	2–6	Intermediate	4–10
High	≥ 7	High	≥ 11
Clinical probability (2 levels)			
PE unlikely	0–4		
PE likely	0–4		

Table 1.
Clinical prediction scores for PE: the revised Geneva score and the Wells score.

In patients with a shock state, besides PE, other causes that should be considered are acute myocardial infarction, cardiac tamponade, acute aortic syndrome, and acute valvular disease. Therefore, echocardiography should be the first choice for differential diagnosis. For unstable patients who cannot be transported to CT immediately, when echocardiography is suggestive (right ventricular overload), the diagnosis of PE can be accepted. After resuscitation, the patient can be transported for a diagnostic CT scan. In stable patients, diagnosis by Christopher's Algorithm (**Figure 17**) [36].

4.4 Histopathology

Pulmonary thromboembolism can form due to stagnation and inflammation or coagulopathy in the large veins in the legs and pelvis. Observed in the pulmonary artery in the left lung on the cut section is massive pulmonary thromboembolism (**Figure 18A**). The "saddle embolus" (**Figure 18B**) is a bridge from the heart across the pulmonary artery and divides into the right and left main pulmonary arteries. This thromboembolism displays a typical gross appearance, irregular surface, and pale tan to white, admixed with dark red areas. It often causes sudden death.

Thrombus layered is typical of a thrombus that forms in a large vein of the pelvis or lower extremity. It has migrated up the inferior vena cava, through the right heart, and into a pulmonary artery (**Figures 18C–23**).

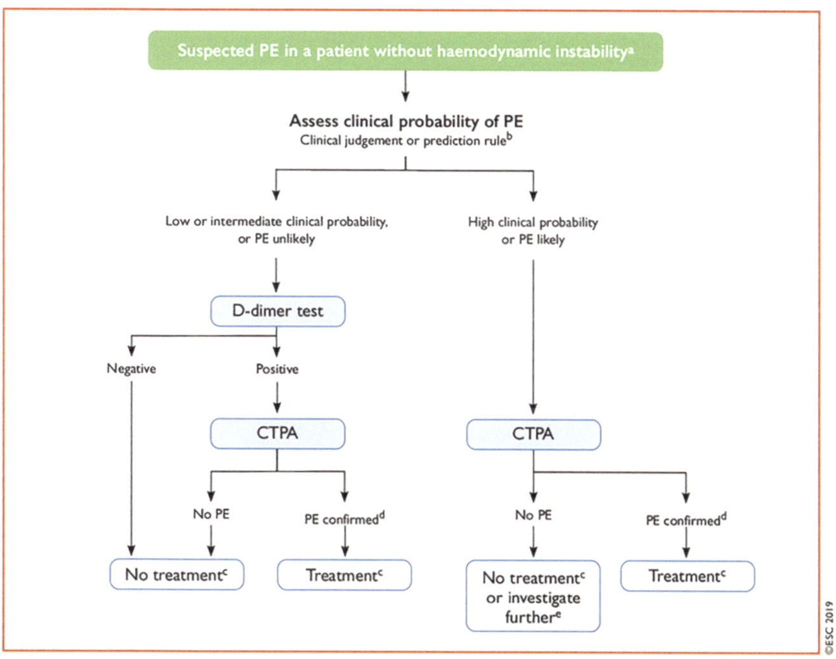

Figure 17.
Christopher's Algorithm.

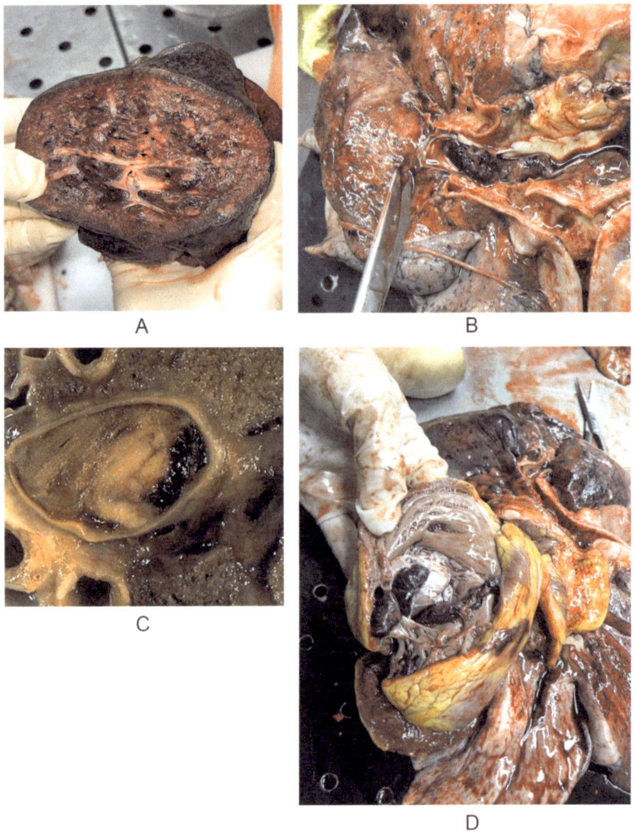

Figure 18.
A: Large pulmonary thromboembolus. B: "Saddle Embolus". C: Thrombus layered. D: PE with right ventricular thrombus.

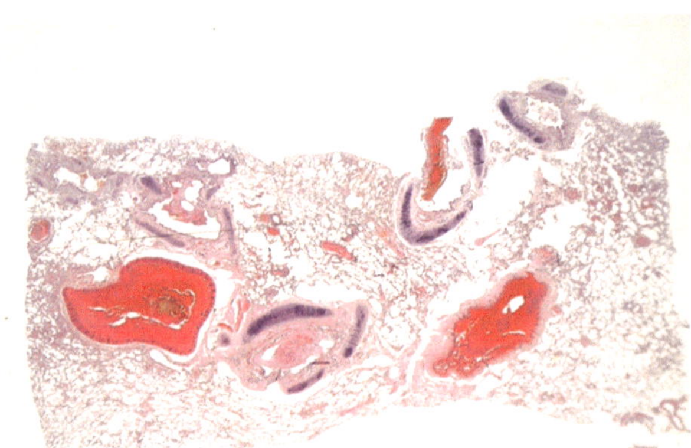

Figure 19.
Thromboembolism is packed into a pulmonary artery.Thromboembolism packs into a pulmonary artery, and thromboembolism forms the organization and dissolution. The interdigitating area of pale pink and red forms the "lines of Zahn" characteristic of a thrombus. These lines represent layers of red cells, platelets, and fibrin laid down in the vessel as the thrombus forms.

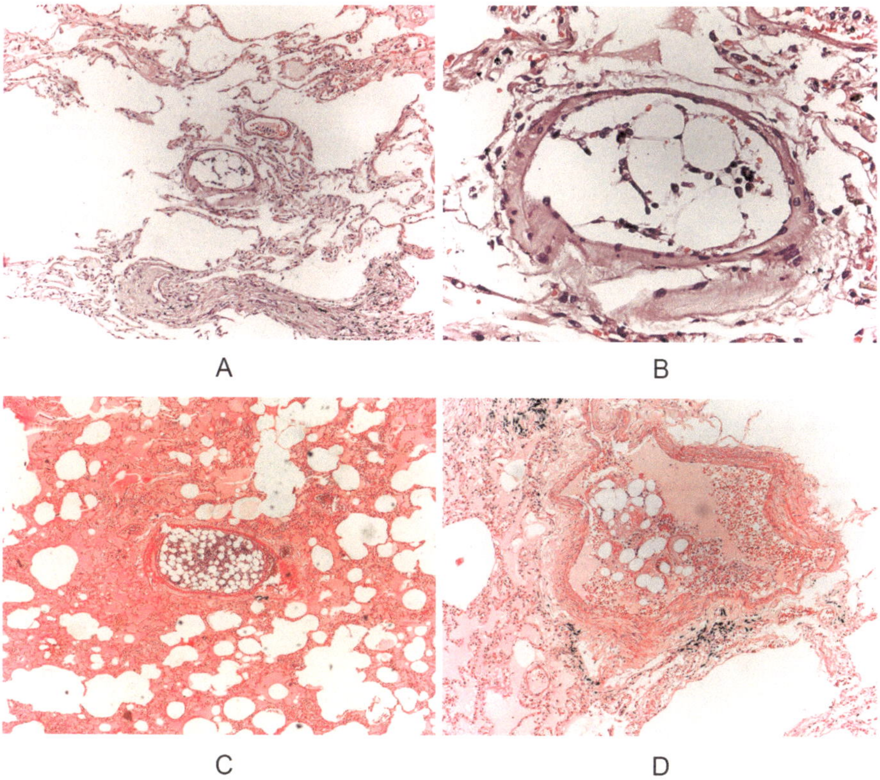

Figure 20.
Fat emboli: The round holes in the vascular spaces of the lung are fat emboli. Fat emboli often occur following trauma with a fracture of long bones. It releases fat globules into the circulation trapped in pulmonary capillaries.

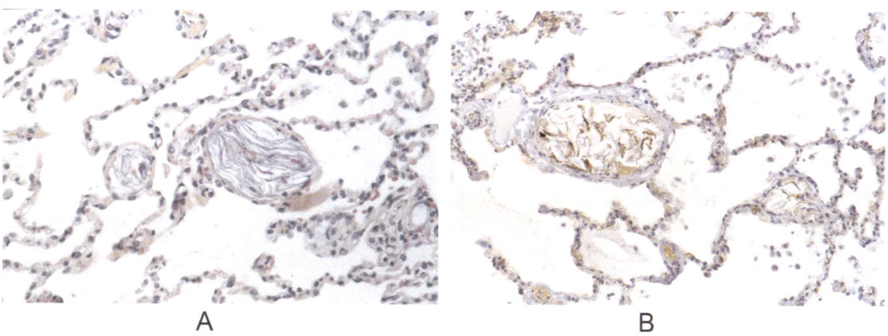

Figure 21.
A: Amniotic fluid embolization (H&E stain). B: Amniotic fluid embolization (Immunohistochemistry CK +) Amniotic fluid embolization: It is an obstetric complication. The pulmonary artery branch is an amniotic fluid embolus with layers of fetal squames, and the outcome is a massive pulmonary embolism.

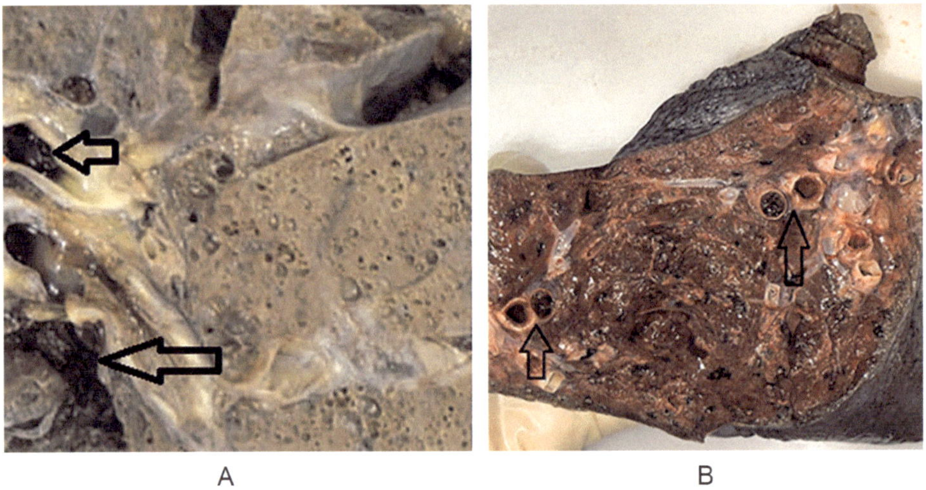

Figure 22.
Pulmonary Arterial Thrombosis due to SARS-CoV-2. Macroscopically: The massive bilateral congestion is grayish-red. The most structural feature is the presence of thrombotic in branches of the pulmonary arteries, varied from focal to extensive in all sizes of the vessels. The bronchial system contains viscous mucus and pleural effusion.

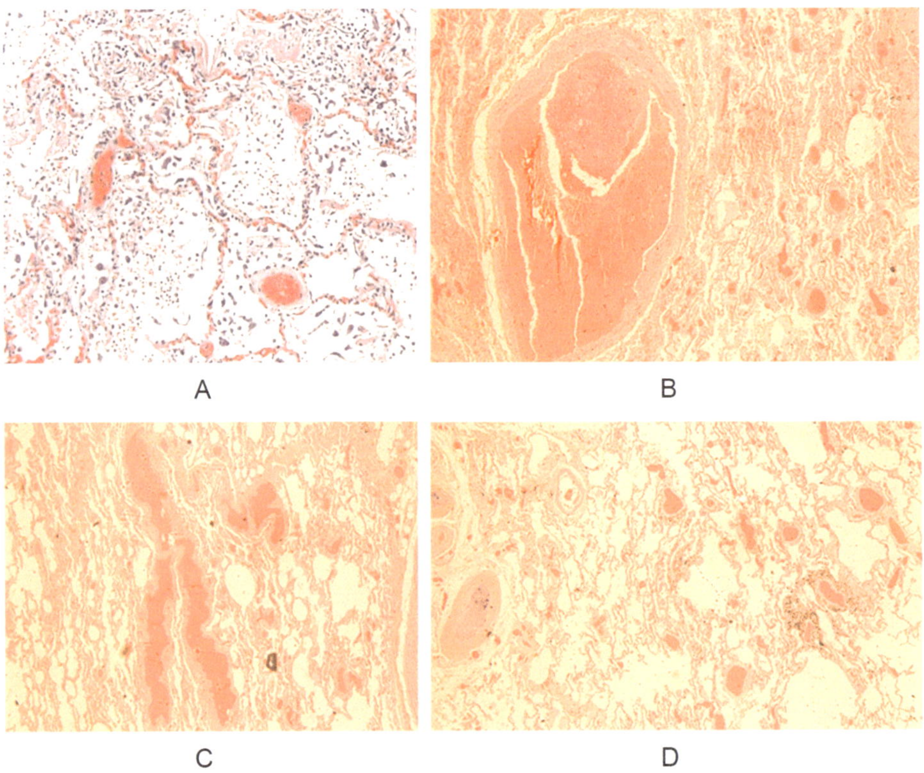

Figure 23.
Pulmonary Arterial Thrombosis due to SARS-CoV-2. Microscopic: Diffuse alveolar damage is a consistent feature of COVID-19, to exudative, proliferative, and fibrotic phases with the alveolar multinucleated giant cells and interstitial and alveolar inflammation. Blood vessels may show fibrinoid necrosis, wall thickening, luminal stenosis, or occlusion. The frequent presence of micro pulmonary thrombosis further supports hypercoagulative status.

DOI: http://dx.doi.org/10.5772/intechopen.110503

Author details

Dang Viet Duc[1]*, Nguyen Thanh Huy[1], Tran Quoc Quy[1] and Nguyen Tat Tho[2]

1 Cardiovascular Intensive Care Unit, Heart Institute, 108 Military Central Hospital, Ha Noi, Viet Nam

2 Military Institute Forensic Medicine, Ha Noi, Viet Nam

*Address all correspondence to: dangvietduc108@gmail.com

References

[1] Knuuti J, Wijns W, Saraste A, Capodanno D, Barbato E, Funck-Brentano C, et al. 2019 ESC Guidelines for the diagnosis and management of chronic coronary syndromes: The Task Force for the diagnosis and management of chronic coronary syndromes of the European Society of Cardiology (ESC). European Heart Journal. 2020;**41**(3): 407-477

[2] Pijls NHJ, Sels JWEM. Functional measurement of coronary stenosis. Journal of the American College of Cardiology. 2012;**59**(12): 1045-1057

[3] Canty JM, Suzuki G. Myocardial perfusion and contraction in acute ischemia and chronic ischemic heart disease. Journal of Molecular and Cellular Cardiology. 2012;**52**(4):822-831

[4] Camici PG, d'Amati G, Rimoldi O. Coronary microvascular dysfunction: Mechanisms and functional assessment. Nature Reviews. Cardiology. 2015;**12**(1): 48-62

[5] Reeh J, Therming CB, Heitmann M, Højberg S, Sørum C, Bech J, et al. Prediction of obstructive coronary artery disease and prognosis in patients with suspected stable angina. European Heart Journal. 2019;**40**(18):1426-1435

[6] Madsen DM, Diederichsen ACP, Hosbond SE, Gerke O, Mickley H. Diagnostic and prognostic value of a careful symptom evaluation and high sensitive troponin in patients with suspected stable angina pectoris without prior cardiovascular disease. Atherosclerosis. 2017;**258**:131-137

[7] Virmani R et al. Lessons from sudden coronary death a comprehensive morphological classification scheme for atherosclerotic lesions. Arteriosclerosis, Thrombosis, and Vascular Biology. 2000;**20**:1262-1275

[8] Collet JP, Thiele H, Barbato E, Barthélémy O, Bauersachs J, Bhatt DL, et al. 2020 ESC Guidelines for the management of acute coronary syndromes in patients presenting without persistent ST-segment elevation: The Task Force for the management of acute coronary syndromes in patients presenting without persistent ST-segment elevation of the European Society of Cardiology (ESC). European Heart Journal. 2021;**42**(14):1289-1367

[9] Heusch G, Gersh BJ. The pathophysiology of acute myocardial infarction and strategies of protection beyond reperfusion: A continual challenge. European Heart Journal. 2017; **38**(11):774-784

[10] Diercks DB, Peacock WF, Hiestand BC, Chen AY, Pollack CV, Kirk JD, et al. Frequency and consequences of recording an electrocardiogram >10 minutes after arrival in an emergency room in non–ST-segment elevation acute coronary syndromes (from the CRUSADE initiative). The American Journal of Cardiology. 2006;**97**(4):437-442

[11] Mandelzweig L, Battler A, Boyko V, Bueno H, Danchin N, Filippatos G, et al. The second Euro Heart Survey on acute coronary syndromes: Characteristics, treatment, and outcome of patients with ACS in Europe and the Mediterranean Basin in 2004. European Heart Journal. 2006;**27**(19):2285-2293

[12] Reichlin T, Twerenbold R, Maushart C, Reiter M, Moehring B, Schaub N, et al. Risk stratification in patients with unstable angina using absolute serial

changes of 3 high-sensitive troponin assays. American Heart Journal. 2013; **165**(3):371-378.e3

[13] Kaier TE, Twerenbold R, Puelacher C, Marjot J, Imambaccus N, Boeddinghaus J, et al. Direct comparison of cardiac myosin-binding protein C with cardiac troponins for the early diagnosis of acute myocardial infarction. Circulation. 2017;**136**(16):1495-1508

[14] Lancellotti P, Price S, Edvardsen T, Cosyns B, Neskovic AN, Dulgheru R, et al. The use of echocardiography in acute cardiovascular care: Recommendations of the European Association of Cardiovascular Imaging and the Acute Cardiovascular Care Association. European Heart Journal of Cardiovascular Imaging. 2015;**16**(2):119-146

[15] Mozaffarian D, Benjamin EJ, Go AS, Arnett DK, Blaha MJ, Cushman M, et al. Heart disease and stroke statistics—2016 update. Circulation. 2016;**133**(4):e38-e360

[16] Seiler C, Stoller M, Pitt B, Meier P. The human coronary collateral circulation: Development and clinical importance. European Heart Journal. 2013;**34**(34):2674-2682

[17] Fishbein MC. The vulnerable and unstable atherosclerotic plaque. Cardiovascular Pathology. 2010;**19**(1): 6-11

[18] Ibanez B, James S, Agewall S, Antunes MJ, Bucciarelli-Ducci C, Bueno H, et al. 2017 ESC Guidelines for the management of acute myocardial infarction in patients presenting with ST-segment elevation: The Task Force for the management of acute myocardial infarction in patients presenting with ST-segment elevation of the European Society of Cardiology (ESC). European Heart Journal. 2018;**39**(2):119-177

[19] Bozkurt B. Current diagnostic and treatment strategies for specific dilated cardiomyopathies: A scientific statement from the American Heart Association. Circulation. 2016;**134**:e579-e646

[20] F. V. DEC GW. Idiopathic dilated cardiomyopathy. The New England Journal of Medicine. 1994;**331**:1564-1575

[21] Schultheiss H-P. Dilated cardiomyopathy. Nature Reviews Disease Primers: Article number: 5. 2019;**32**

[22] Elliott P. Diagnosis and management of dilated cardiomyopathy. Cardiomyopathy. 2000;**84**:106-106

[23] Ommen SR, Mital S, et al. 2020 AHA/ACC guideline for the diagnosis and treatment of patients with hypertrophic cardiomyopathy. Circulation. 2020;**142**:e558-e631

[24] Davies MW. Hypertrophic cardiomyopathy-pathology and pathogenesis. Histopathology. 1995;**26**: 493-500

[25] Snir W. Exercise in hypertrophic cardiomyopathy: Restrict or rethink. American Journal of Physiology. 2021; **2021**

[26] Finocchiaro G. The electrocardiogram in the diagnosis and management of patients with hypertrophic cardiomyopathy. Heart Rhythm. 2020;**17**(1):142-151

[27] Muchtar E. Restrictive cardiomyopathy genetics, pathogenesis, clinical manifestations, diagnosis, and therapy. Circulation Research. 2017;**121**: 819-837

[28] B. S. (99m)Tc-pyrophosphate scintigraphy for differentiating light-chain cardiac amyloidosis from the

transthyretin-related familial and senile cardiac amyloidoses. Circulation. Cardiovascular Imaging. 2013;**6**:195-201

[29] Tapson VF. Acute pulmonary embolism. New England Journal of Medicine. 2008;**358**:1037-1052

[30] Tapson VF. Pulmonary Embolism. Fuster and Hurst's The Heart. 2022. p. 15e. ISBN 978-1-264-25756-0

[31] Ceriani E et al. Clinical prediction rules for pulmonary embolism: A systematic review and meta-analysis. Journal of Thrombosis and Haemostasis. 2010;**8**(5):957-970

[32] Manier G. Determinants of hypoxemia during the acute phase of pulmonary embolism in humans. The American Review of Respiratory Disease. 1985;**132**(02):332-338

[33] Konstantinides SV et al. ESC Guidelines for the diagnosis and management of acute pulmonary embolism developed in collaboration with the European Respiratory Society (ERS). European Respiratory Journal. 2019;**54**:1901647

[34] Olsson OK et al. Chronic thromboembolic pulmonary hypertension. Deutsches Ärzteblatt International. 2014;**111**:856-862

[35] Riedel M. Acute pulmonary embolism: Pathophysiology, clinical presentation, and diagnosis. Heart. 2001; **85**:229-240

[36] Belle V et al. Effectiveness of managing suspected pulmonary embolism using an algorithm combining clinical probability, D-dimer testing, and computed tomography. JAMA. 2006;**295** (2):172-179

Chapter 3

Molecular Histopathology of Mammary Carcinogenesis as Approach to Cancer Prediction and Prevention

Dyah Ayu Oktavianie A. Pratama

Abstract

Breast/mammary cancer is the most frequent type of cancer and the leading cause of cancer deaths in humans and animals worldwide. The incidence of mammary cancer is continuously increasing worldwide. This increasing trend is attributed partly to the little information on the early changes occurring during mammary gland carcinogenesis. The lack of molecular information on mammary carcinogenesis has impeded the identification of clinically relevant tumor markers beyond histopathology and the introduction of new therapeutic concepts. Numerous factors, molecular and cellular pathways are involved in mammary tumor development and carcinogenesis. To characterize some of the early molecular changes of mammary carcinogenesis, mammary cancer was induced in female rats using the environmental carcinogen 7,12 dimethylbenz (α) anthracene (DMBA) combined with estrogen. Analysis of histopathological alterations in the tissue can observe the process of mammary cancer development. At the molecular level, some genes act as functional components in regulating cancer development, including tumor suppressor genes, oncogenes, and DNA repair genes. In this chapter, the histopathological alterations and the advanced of molecular histopathology stages of breast cancer progression are mainly discussed, including on animal models induced by DMBA-estrogen combination as an effort for cancer prediction and prevention.

Keywords: molecular histopathology, protein markers, mammary cancer, carcinogenesis, DMBA

1. Introduction

Mammary cancer is one of the most common malignancies neoplasms and the leading cause of mortality that affects female dogs and cats worldwide. It is similar to human breast cancer as cancer initially arises from the mammary gland. In humans, it is commonly known as breast cancer since the anatomical location which is at the breast [1]. There are approximately 54,000 and 207,000 new cases of *in situ* and invasive breast carcinoma in humans [2]. Breast cancer also represents the highest cancer mortality rates in women across the globe [3]. Mammary cancer can also occur in animals, including companion animals such as female dogs over six years of age. The incidence of mammary tumors in dogs is around 46.79%, while other tumors are about 53.21% [4]. In animals, female dogs and cats have a high prevalence of mammary cancer, which account for 52% and 17%, respectively [1].

Many factors like molecular and cellular pathways are believed to be involved in mammary gland development and carcinogenesis [5, 6]. Factors that can cause breast/mammary cancer include the loss of tumor suppressors, the presence of abnormal estrogenic activity, and the presence of carcinogens or cancer-causing agents that can cause genetic mutations [7]. Mammary cancers that arise in animals are similar to human breast cancers in clinical, histopathological, and molecular features. For this reason, studies on animal models of mammary cancer are highly relevant to correlate prognosis and therapeutic value prior to inclusion in clinical trials [1]. Genetic mutagens from cancer-causing carcinogens or exposure to radiation have led researchers to develop breast cancer in animal models containing carcinogens. Recently, the prevention of breast cancer has received much attention. Several of the established experimental animal models of mammary cancer offer a wide range of options for studying environmental and genetic factors and therapeutics associated with breast cancer. Using a chemical-induced rat mammary cancer model, it can be concluded that the histopathological changes in rat mammary cancer are similar to those in humans [8].

One substance that is known to be carcinogenic is 7,12-dimethylbenz(α) anthracene (DMBA), which is mutagenic, teratogenic, carcinogenic, cytotoxic, and immunosuppressive. DMBA is a synthetic polycyclic aromatic hydrocarbon. Researchers have concluded that DMBA is a potential carcinogen and may act on multiple sites, including the skin [9], mammary glands [10], oral cavity [11], and pancreas [12]. The risk of developing mammary cancer may also be influenced by the role of estrogen. Estrogen is a potent stimulator of mammary epithelial cell proliferation. The most potent and abundant estrogen in the body is 17β-estradiol (E2) [13]. Cancer cells can transform, proliferate, and metastasize, thus altering the histopathological appearance of the cells. Studies have shown that breast/mammary cancer development is a multi-step process that progresses from normal to generalized hyperplasia, atypical hyperplasia, carcinoma *in situ*, and finally the invasive stage of cancer. Continuing advances in understanding the molecular pathology of breast cancer progression have contributed to the discovery of new pathway-specific targeted therapies, and with the advent of such potent therapeutics, now molecular-based "patient-specific" is an increasing need for treatment plans. Insights gained from studying the molecular pathology of mammary cancer progression in animal models, and the integration and translation of these insights into the clinical setting, have the potential to further reduce breast/mammary cancer morbidity and mortality.

In this chapter, we describe the histopathological alterations in a Sprague–Dawley (SD) rats mammary cancer model induced by the combination of 7,12-dimethylbenz (a) anthracene (DMBA) and estrogen and molecular histopathology pattern of some protein markers of mammary carcinogenesis. This chapter also describes the theoretical classification of breast cancer based on histopathology and molecular histopathology. Understanding correlations between animal mammary cancer and human breast cancer can contribute to further investigation for treatment and prevention. Similar to the structure of human breast cancer, the rat mammary gland is also known to have a terminal duct-lobular unit (TDLU). The animal model mammary cancer induced by DMBA closely resembles human breast cancer originating from TDLU, and the histopathological changes and premalignant to malignant progression are similar to those of human breast cancer [8]. Therefore, DMBA-induced mammary cancer in rats is a valuable tool for investigating the mechanisms of pathogenesis and development of human breast cancer and its prevention.

2. Histopathological alterations of the mammary gland during carcinogenesis in rats induced by DMBA-estrogen combination

The mammary gland is a hormone-dependent organ that is influenced by steroid hormones secreted by the ovary. It was previously known that DMBA induces mammary cancer under hormonal conditions in the presence of adequate levels of estrogen. Estrogen stimulates ductal growth, epithelial hyperplasia, and the development of connective tissue-enclosed ducts and lobules, increasing the number of progestogen receptors in mammary cells, and promoting lobular acinar development has been shown in numerous studies [8].

Histopathological analysis plays an important role in tumor diagnosis and research. Although the histopathological features of the human breast cancer are well known, details about the mechanisms involved in breast cancer and the associated histomorphology alterations are still unclear. The morphological features of rat mammary carcinoma are similar to those of human breast carcinoma. In this study, histopathological observation of a rat mammary cancer model induced by the DMBA-estrogen combination was performed using the Hematoxylin–Eosin (HE) staining method (**Figure 1**).

7,12-Dimethylbenz(α)anthracene (DMBA), a toxic tumor-inducing agent that has been proven in animal models, has also been reported to induce human breast cancer [14]. It is mainly reported to induce the formation of terminal ductal lesions, and induce ductal epithelial cell hyperplasia, atypical hyperplasia, and subsequent ductal changes [8].

Our study also confirmed that many types of mammary gland lesions that occurred in rats induced by DMBA and estrogen combination are similar to lesions in human breast cancer. As a result of the induction of DMBA, in the treatment group, alveolar epithelial cells have dysplasia, and their shape and structure have changed compared with control group. The alveolar cells are no longer round, their arrangement is irregular, and there is a change in the shape of the epithelial cells. The normal alveolar epithelial cells are cuboid in layers (**Figure 1A**). The dysplasia found in the alveoli indicates that there has been a neoplastic or cancerous process in the breast. In the treatment group, hyper-chromatin is also found in the cell nucleus so that it looks darker (**Figure 1B**). The mammary duct is normally covered by a layer of epithelial cells and the ductal lumen is empty (**Figure 1C**). The treatment group showed a hyperplasia or proliferation of epithelial cells from the surface of the duct to the lumen of the duct (**Figure 1D**). According to Young et al., tissue in the mammary or stroma is in the form of connective tissue and fatty tissue that surrounds the lobes (**Figure 1E**). In treatment group, new cancer cells form new epithelial cell clusters that had spread to the surrounding tissue (**Figure 1F**).

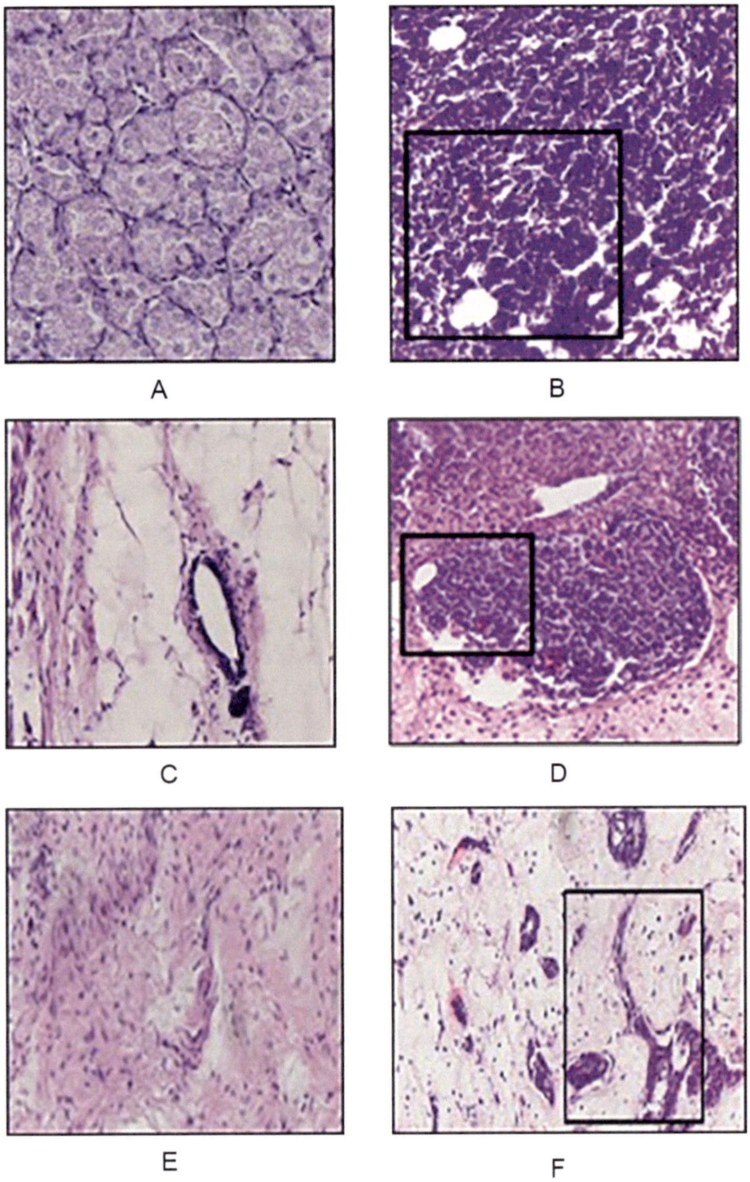

Figure 1.
Histopathological alterations in rat mammary cancer model induced by DMBA-estrogen combination. Mammary alveolar on control group shows a normal morphology (a). The formation of neoplastic cell on mammary alveolar is shown with dysplasia of alveolar epithelial cell (B). The mammary duct in control group is normally covered by a layer of epithelial cells and the ductal lumen is empty (C). Hyperplasia of ductal epithelial cell to basement membrane (D). Stroma in the form of connective tissue and fatty tissue that surrounds the lobes (E). Invasion of cancer cell to mammary stroma (F) (HE, original magnification ×400).

According to Feng et al. [8], the carcinogen DMBA and hormone intervention can cause the presence of pre-malignant lesions such as usual ductal hyperplasia (UDH), atypical ductal hyperplasia (ADH), and ductal carcinoma in situ (DCIS) and invasive ductal carcinoma (IDC) (**Figure 2**) [15]. The UDH sample showed proliferative cells that were arranged in a mixed and disorderly pattern (**Figure 2A**). In the ADH samples, the ductal epithelial cells were bigger than

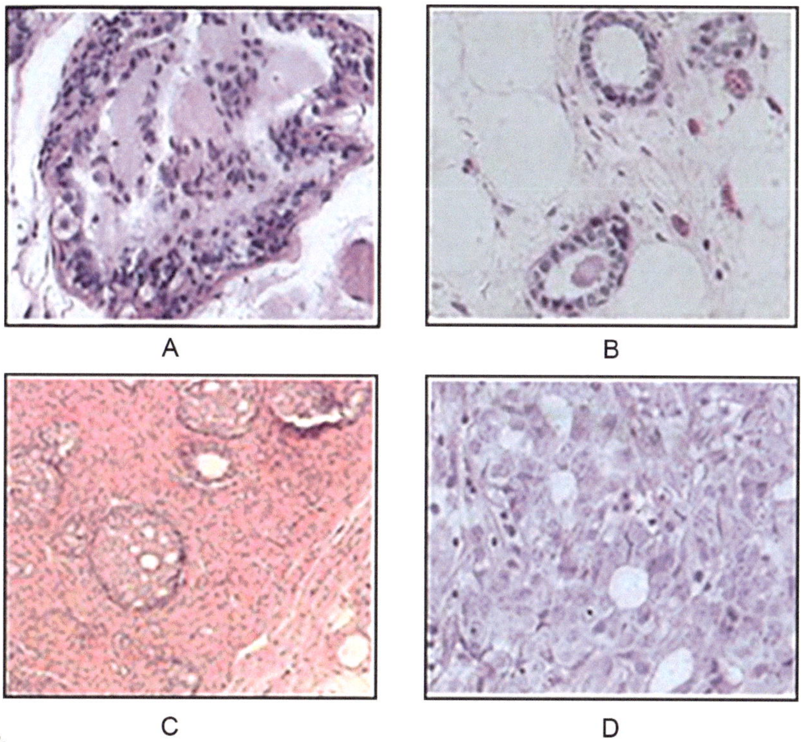

Figure 2.
Histopathological changes in breast tissue in the SD rat model. UDH tissue showed proliferative cells in a mixed and disorderly pattern (a). ADH tissue showed that the ductal epithelial cells were larger than normal cells and had an increased cytoplasm-nucleus ratio (B). DCIS tissue showed that the lumen of the duct was filled with atypical proliferative cells (C). IDC tissue showed that the proliferative cells (D) (HE, original magnification ×400). Adapted from Feng et al. [8].

normal cells and had an increased cytoplasm-nucleus ratio (**Figure 2B**). In the DCIS sample, the lumen of the duct was filled with atypical proliferative cells that formed a cribriform (**Figure 2C**). Further, proliferative tumor cells were observed to damage the basement membrane and then infiltrate into the fibrous connective tissue, namely IDC (**Figure 2D**).

3. Histopathological classification of mammary cancer

The animal mammary cancer classification is adapted from the breast cancer classification system. Breast cancer classification is based on pathology and molecular biology [16, 17]. To study the breast/mammary cancer morphology, it is necessary to understand whether the tumor is confined to the epithelial component of the breast, invades the surrounding stroma, or develops in the ducts or lobes of the mammary gland [3]. In the practice of histopathology, cell type features, number of cells, type and location of secretion, immunohistochemical profile, and structural features, in addition to their subclassification, are used to determine whether the tumors are ductal or lobular.

The most common special types of breast cancer (**Figure 3**) according to Nascimento and Otoni [3] include the following:

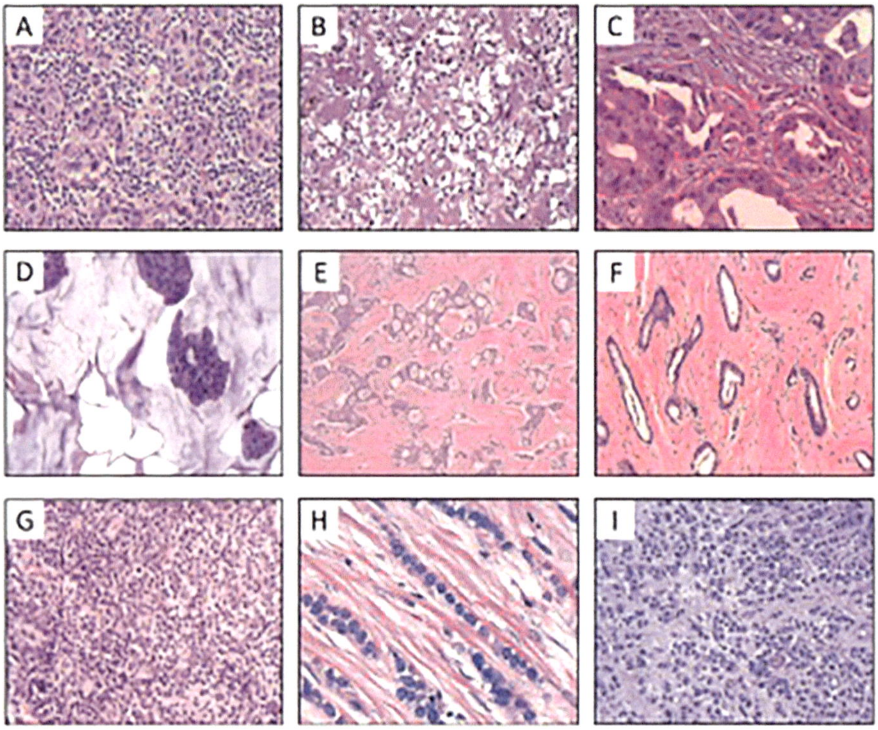

Figure 3.
The morphological classification of the main subtypes of invasive breast carcinomas. (A) Medullary carcinoma; (B) metaplastic carcinoma; (C) apocrine carcinoma; (D) mucinous carcinoma; (E) cribriform carcinoma; (F) tubular carcinoma; (G) neuroendocrine carcinoma; (H) classic lobular carcinoma; and (I) pleomorphic lobular carcinoma (adapted from Nascimento and Otoni, [3]).

3.1 Invasive ductal carcinoma non-specific type (IDC-NST)

The most common histological subtype in about 40–75% all invasive breast carcinoma. The morphology of tumor cells is pleomorphic, with protruding nucleoli and numerous mitoses.

3.2 Medullary carcinoma

Special subtype of invasive breast carcinoma, responsible for approximately 5% of all cases, is associated with mutations in BRCA-1 germline. The microscopic morphology is marked with well-circumscribed carcinoma, composed of large and pleomorphic tumor cells, frequent mitotic figures, and prominent lymphoplasmacytic infiltrate (**Figure 3A**). Other commonly seen features are spindle cell metaplasia and giant tumor cells.

3.3 Metaplastic carcinoma

This subtype is characterized by the dominant component of metaplastic differentiation, representing approximately 1% of all cases. Morphologically marked with a poorly differentiated heterogeneous tumor that contains ductal carcinoma cells mixed with other histological elements, such as squamous cells, spindle cells or other mesenchymal differentiation (chondroid cells, bone cells, and myoepithelial cells) (**Figure 3B**).

3.4 Apocrine carcinoma

This subtype constitutes about 1–4% of all cases, with prominent apocrine differentiation comprising at least 90% of tumor cells, microscopically marked with large tumor cells with an abundant granular eosinophilic cytoplasm and prominent nucleoli. In addition, bizarre tumor cells with multi-lobulated nuclei can also be observed (**Figure 3C**).

3.5 Mucinous carcinoma

This is a special subtype of breast cancer, also known as colloid, gelatinous, mucous, and mucoid carcinoma, responsible for 2% of all newly diagnosed cases. Morphologically, these tumors have abundant amounts of extracellular mucin, surrounding small clusters of tumor cells with different growth patterns and mild nuclear atypia (**Figure 3D**).

3.6 Cribriform carcinoma

Special subtype of breast cancer constitutes about 1–3.5% of all breast cancer cases. Microscopically marked with islands of uniform tumor cells, with low grade atypia, cribriform appearance in 90% of the tumor is often associated with DCIS without well-defined stromal invasion (**Figure 3E**).

3.7 Tubular carcinoma

This subtype is characterized by the proliferation of prominent tubules, which can be angled, oval, or elongated, with a disorganized disposition and open lumen covered by a single layer of epithelium, without presentation of necrosis and mitosis (**Figure 3F**).

3.8 Neuroendocrine carcinoma

It accounts for about 0.5–5% of all breast cancer cases. Morphological appearance shows an infiltrative growth pattern with solid aggregates of tumor cells arranged in an alveolar, trabecular, or rosette-like pattern, and a peripheral palisade may also be observed. Tumor cells vary in size and generally have an eosinophilic granular cytoplasm (**Figure 3G**).

3.9 Invasive lobular carcinoma

This subtype is the second largest biologically distinct carcinoma, accounting for approximately 5–15% of all newly breast cancer cases. The classic morphology of ILC is characterized by the presence of small tumor cells with mild atypia, evenly distributed over the stroma in a concentric pattern (**Figure 3H**).

Histology types of induced breast cancer using DMBA are generally papillary carcinoma and cribriform carcinoma [18, 19].

4. The mechanism of molecular carcinogenesis

Studies of neoplastic disease development, and cellular and molecular mechanisms have identified many individual molecules and signaling pathways, especially in humans and experimental animals. Despite the widely accepted notion that cancer results from defective genes (mainly oncogenes and tumor suppressor genes), new principles, pathways, and molecules are emerging that are responsible for the neoplastic transformation of cells. It remains to be found as an essential factor in metastatic malignant progression and fatal outcomes. Certain functional groups of molecules are involved in different stages of tumor progression and metastasis, including mediators of apoptosis and DNA repair, oncogenes and tumor suppressors, adhesion molecules, mediators of angiogenesis, and markers of circulating tumor cells [20].

4.1 Tumor growth: proto-oncogenes and oncogenes

Neoplastic growth of mammary tissue is marked by increased cell proliferation compared to non-neoplastic mammary epithelium. Mammary tumor cells have overexpression of growth-promoting gene products (proto-oncogenes), decreased expression levels, or functional activity of growth-inhibiting gene products (tumor suppressors) involved in promoting growth. Proto-oncogenes are directly involved in cell cycle progression, such as members of cell cycle checkpoints (cyclins, cyclin-dependent kinases [CDK], retinoblastoma proteins), and indirectly involved in cell cycle progression. Any of the members of the molecular network induces growth factor receptor pathway. Growth factor signaling can have both growth-stimulatory and growth-inhibitory effects on breast tumors. Some of the growth-promoting signaling pathways in breast tumors are epidermal growth factor 2 (ERBB2) and epidermal growth factor 1 (EGFR1). Other than EGFR, metastatic canine mammary carcinomas show decreased expression of several transmembrane growth factor receptors compared to non-metastatic carcinomas or normal glands, such as members of the transforming growth factor beta receptor (TGFBR), fibroblast growth factor receptor (FGFR), and growth hormone receptor (GHR).

Proteomic analyses comparing metastatic and non-metastatic simple breast cancer identified an alteration in expression patterns of several growth-promoting and proliferation-related genes. These genes include the Ran/TC4-binding protein (RANBP1), which is involved in spindle cell assembly, the protein elongation factor 1δ (EEF1D), which is potentially involved in neoplastic transformation and carcinogenesis, and the proliferation nuclear antigen (PCNA), which is a requirement for DNA replication.

4.2 Loss of growth inhibition: tumor suppressors

Dysregulated cell proliferation in non-neoplastic cells is tightly regulated by multiple molecular pathways, including cell cycle checkpoints and various tumor suppressors. Malignant breast tumors have an increased proportion of cells with active cell cycle progression, as shown by Ki67 and PCNA immunohistochemistry. One of the most characterized tumor suppressors and growth inhibitors is p53. This protein is activated by multiple triggers, including oxidative stress and DNA damage, leading to irreversible cell cycle arrest. Cell cycle arrest by p53 is mediated by increased transcription of p21, an inhibitor of cyclin E/Cdk2, at the G1-to-M cell cycle transition checkpoint. The increased expression of p21 in metastatic breast tumors may be an attempt by p53 induction to inhibit cell cycle progression, which fails in the majority of tumor cells. Like p21, p27 regulates cell cycle progression through interaction with cyclin E/Cdk2 or cyclin D/Cdk4. Moreover, p27 expression is decreased in metastatic carcinoma and its metastases, as well as in adenomas, suggesting that loss of p27 expression occurs early in malignant transformation of mammary epithelium.

The phosphatase and tensin homolog (PTEN) appears to be another interesting tumor suppressor with prognostic relevance for mammary tumors. PTEN reduces cell proliferation but is involved in apoptosis induction and cell adhesion.

4.3 Cell proliferation and prognosis

Increased cell proliferation is a clear feature of malignant mammary tumors. Three molecular markers that have been successfully used to measure proliferative activity through histological methods are PCNA, Ki67, and AgNOR.

PCNA is present in the cell nucleus and acts as a cofactor for the DNA polymerase δ, thus increasing DNA replication. PCNA concentrations peak during the G1 and S phases of the cell cycle but are also found in cells that have recently completed the M phase due to its long half-life of 8–20 hours. Ki67 is a heterodimeric protein with peak expression during the M phase of the cell cycle. A nuclear organizer region (NOR) is a chromosomal segment involved in ribosome biogenesis. They are composed of an argyrophilic protein and thus AgNOR that co-localizes with the nucleolar ribosomal DNA loop. The rearrangement of these loops is directly related to cell proliferative activity.

4.4 Apoptosis: loss of the emergency switch

In non-neoplastic cells, genetic and metabolic imbalances that can lead to malignant transformation are prevented by multiple molecular mechanisms that ultimately lead to apoptosis or programmed cell death. Severe DNA damage under physiological conditions; imprecise DNA replication; dysregulation of cell cycle progression; hypoxic stress is a typical event that causes the activation of pro-apoptotic pathways or the suppression of anti-apoptotic pathways and molecules.

One of the central regulators in the early stages of apoptosis induction is the tumor suppressor p53. In stressed cells or severe DNA damage, activated p53 accumulates within the cell and leads to cell cycle arrest. This either activates the DNA damage response or, in the case of irreparable DNA damage, induces apoptosis *via* the activation of pro-apoptotic proteins (bax). Bax activation ultimately leads to the activation of apoptosis-associated initiators, cysteine peptidases (caspases). Several p53 mutations have been identified in breast tumor cases. Furthermore, p53 mRNA and protein expression data in malignant tumors report differently between normal and elevated expressions compared to benign tumors or normal glands. Proteins involved in downstream signaling of p53 and other triggers of apoptosis have been extensively analyzed. In some studies, breast cancers showed increased or unchanged expression of anti-apoptotic proteins (BCL2, BCLX, SFRP2), but decreased expression of pro-apoptotic proteins (BAX, caspase-8, caspase-9).

Rapid growth of malignant tumors causes cytotoxic stress such as hypoxia and nutritional deficiencies. As a result, tumor cells accumulate misfolded proteins in the endoplasmic reticulum, ultimately inducing apoptosis and reducing cell viability.

4.5 DNA repair: failure of the DNA quality management

Carcinogens can initially cause DNA damage, but later stages of cancer progression exhibit chromosomal instability. Aberrant cell proliferation caused by mutations activating proto-oncogenes or inactivation of tumor suppressors can continuously induce DNA replication stress. Chronic hypoxia and/or cycles of hypoxia and reoxygenation contribute to genomic instability. This is not unique to tumor cells, but is fairly common in non-tumor cells in the body at any time. In consequence of the wide variety of DNA damage forms, mammalian cells possess multiple DNA repair tools, including non-homologous termination; homologous recombination; base excision repair; nucleotide excision repair; mismatch repair; and transregion synthesis. Mutations or epigenetic inactivation of DNA repair genes accumulate during tumor progression, causing alterations in DNA repair mechanisms and accelerating malignant progression by increasing mutation rates.

In human breast cancer, approximately 5–10% are considered hereditary and associated with germline mutations in breast cancer susceptibility genes 1 and 2 (BRCA1 and BRCA2) that play a role in maintaining genomic stability by functioning as a DNA damage sensor and inducer of the DNA repair response. Several single-nucleotide polymorphisms in the BRCA1 and BRCA2 genomic sequences have been identified in breast tumor cases. In immunohistochemical patterns, malignant breast tumors show decreased nuclear expression and increased cytoplasmic expression of the BRCA1 protein. BRCA-mediated DNA repair is accomplished through the interaction and activation of BRCA1 and BRCA2 with DNA repair proteins, such as RAD51 that increases in metastatic malignant tumor, and p53 which is activated after the identification of DNA damage and which induces cell cycle arrest to allow either DNA repair or apoptosis.

4.6 Cell adhesion molecules

The multicellular organisms' development requires a dynamic and well-coordinated intercellular adhesion system. During various physiological and pathological processes such as tissue development, cell growth, differentiation, embryogenesis, immune response, tumor development, and progression, cell junctions are reorganized and regulated by a network of protein complexes. During carcinogenesis, this complex network of cell–cell contacts is altered, leading to disruption of barriers that facilitate cancer progression and metastasis. Alterations in the expression or function of adhesion molecules at tight, adherens, and gap junctions are critical to tumor progression, including detachment of tumor cells from the primary site, vascular invasion, extravasation into distant target organs, and the formation of metastases. Cell adhesion molecules involved in tumorigenesis include cadherins and catenins, sialylated antigens, claudins, connexins, CD44, HEPACAM1, and HEPACAM2.

4.7 Angiogenesis

Angiogenesis is the formation of new capillaries from pre-existing blood vessels in adults. It is induced in several physiological and pathological (wound healing) non-neoplastic conditions and has profound implications for tumor growth and metastasis. These newly formed blood vessels within the tumor have three main functions; provide nutrients and oxygen to the rapidly growing tumor mass; remove metabolites; and provide an easily accessible exit for metastatic tumor cells entering the systemic circulation.

One of the most important and well-studied stimulators of angiogenesis in malignant tumors is the vascular endothelial growth factor (VEGF) family of proteins. VEGF protein is synthesized and localized in cytoplasmic granules of neoplastic epithelial, endothelial, and stromal cells, suggesting that both autocrine and paracrine signaling induce proliferation of endothelial buds. Besides VEGF, angiopoietins (ANG) 1 and 2 are the only other angiogenic factors analyzed immunohistochemically in malignancies.

Molecular subtypes	**Luminal A**	**Luminal B**		**HER2+**	**TN**
		HER2-	**HER2+**		
Biomarkers	ER+	ER+	ER+	ER−	ER−
	PR+	PR−	PR−/+	PR−	PR−
	HER2−	HER2−	HER2+	HER2+	HER2−
	Ki67low	Ki67high	Ki67low/high	Ki67high	Ki67high
Frequency of cases (%)	40–50	20–30		15–20	10–20
Histological grade	Well differentiated (Grade I)	Moderately differentiated (Grade II)		Little differentiated (Grade III)	Little differentiated (Grade III)
Prognosis	Good	Intermediate		Poor	Poor
Response to therapies	Endocrine	Endocrine Chemotherapy	Endocrine Chemotherapy Target therapy	Target therapy Chemotherapy	Chemotherapy PARP Inhibitors

(Source: Nascimento and Otoni: Histological and molecular classification of breast cancer: what do we know? Copyright © 2020 Brazilian Society of Mastology. All rights reserved).

Table 1.
Molecular histopathology classification of breast cancer.

5. The molecular histopathology classification of breast cancer

In the era of modern medicine, it is not enough to predict the actual behavior of breast tumor pathophysiology based on morphological classification and clinico-pathological parameters alone [19]. Many studies have therefore focused on analyzing the molecular patterns of breast cancer to classify these tumors into classes or entities to aid clinical management. According to Perou et al. (2003), breast cancer is molecularly classified based on similarity of gene expression profiles. Based on extensive studies of gene expression profiles, four clinically relevant molecular subtypes have been identified, including Luminal A, Luminal B, enriched HER2 (HER2+), and Triple Negative (TN). The gene clusters primarily responsible for segregating the molecular subtypes of breast cancer are estrogen receptor (ER), progesterone receptor (PR), human epidermal growth factor receptor 2 (HER2), and cell growth regulator (Ki-67). An immunohistochemistry (IHC) panel using these four biomarkers (ER/PR/HER2/Ki-67) was considered efficient and important in stratifying these molecular entities (**Table 1**).

The use of molecular subtyping enables the possibility of stratifying the neoplasm in different entities that may require specific treatments and different monitoring strategies, in addition to a better understanding of the pathophysiological pattern and clinical prognosis.

6. Conclusion

A series of morphological changes have been observed in the mammary glands of DMBA-estrogen-treated rats. These changes are taken to be representative of the multi-step process that occurs on the development of mammary cancer. Our study also confirmed that many types of mammary gland lesions that occurred in rats induced by DMBA and estrogen combination are similar to lesions in human breast cancer, and being adapted also for histopathological classification. Analysis of histopathology and molecular histopathology classification has a high potential implication for diagnosis, prognosis, and drug targets, and predict the therapeutic response.

Acknowledgements

The authors would like to thank the Faculty of Veterinary Medicine, Universitas Brawijaya for the provision of facilities that allows the writing of this manuscript.

Conflict of interest

The authors declare there is no conflict of interest related to the preparation of this manuscript.

Author details

Dyah Ayu Oktavianie A. Pratama
Laboratory of Anatomical Pathology, Faculty of Veterinary Medicine, Brawijaya University, Malang, East Java, Indonesia

*Address all correspondence to: dyah_ayu@ub.ac.id

References

[1] Nordin ML, Osman AY, Shaari R, Arshad MM, Kadir AA, Reduan MFH. Recent overview of mammary cancer in dogs and cats: Classification, risk factors and future perspectives for treatment. IOSR Journal of Agriculture and Veterinary Science (IOSR-JAVS). 2017;**10**(8):64-69. DOI: 10.9790/2380-1008026469

[2] Bombonati A, Sgroi DC. The molecular pathology of breast cancer progression. The Journal of Pathology. 2011;**223**(2):307-317. DOI: 10.1002/path.2808

[3] Nascimento RGD, Otoni KM. Review article: Histological and molecular classification of breast cancer: What do we know? Mastology. 2020;**30**:e20200024. DOI: 10.29289/25945394202020200024

[4] Itoh T, Uchida K, Ishikawa K, Kushima K, Kushima E, Tamada H, et al. Clinicopathological survey of 101 canine mammary gland tumors: Differences between small – Breed dogs and others. The Journal of Veterinary Medical Science. 2005;**67**(3):345-347. DOI: 10.1292/jvms.67.345

[5] Cocola C, Sanzone S, Astigiano S, Pelucchi P, Piscitelli E, Vilardo L, et al. A rat mammary gland cancer cell with stem cell properties of self- renewal and muti-lineage differentiation. Cytotechnology. 2008;**58**:25-32. DOI: 10.1007/s10616-008-9173-9

[6] Kariagina A, Xie J, Leipprandt JR, Haslam SZ. Amphiregulin mediates estrogen, progester- one, and EGFR signaling in the normal rat mammary gland and in hormone-dependent rat mammary cancers. Horm Cancer. 2010;**1**:229-244. DOI: 10.1007/s12672-010-0048-0

[7] Feng Y, Spezia M, Huang S, Yuan C, Zeng Z, Zhang L, et al. Breast cancer development and progression: Risk factors, cancer stem cells, signaling pathways, genomics, and molecular pathogenesis. Genes & Diseases. 2018;**5**:77-106. DOI: 10.1016/j.gendis.2018.05.001

[8] Feng M, Feng C, Yu Z, Fu Q, Ma Z, Wang F, et al. Histopathological alterations during breast carcinogenesis in a rat model induced by 7,12-Dimethylbenz (a) anthracene and estrogen-progestogen combinations. International Journal of Clinical and Experimental Medicine. 2015;**8**(1):346-357

[9] Manoharan S, Selvan MV. Chemo-preventive potential of geraniol in 7,12-dimethylbenz (a) anthracene (DMBA) induced skin carcinogenesis in Swiss albino mice. Journal of Environmental Biology. 2012;**33**:255-260

[10] Pugalendhi P, Manoharan S, Suresh K, Baskaran N. Genistein and daidzein, in combination, protect cellular integrity during 7,12 dimethylbenz [a] anthracene (DMBA) induced mammary carcinogenesis in Sprague-Dawley rats. African Journal of Traditional, Complementary, and Alternative Medicines. 2011;**8**(2):91-97. DOI: 10.4314/ajtcam.v8i2.63196

[11] Vidya Priyadarsini R, Kumar N, Khan I, Thiyagarajan P, Kondaiah P, Nagini S. Gene expression signature of DMBA-induced hamster buccal pouch carcinomas: Modulation by chlorophyllin and ellagic acid. PLoS One. 2012;**7**(4):e34628. DOI: 10.1371/journal.pone.0034628

[12] Kimura K, Satoh K, Kanno A, Hamada S, Hirota M, Endoh M, et al.

Activation of notch signaling in tumorigenesis of experimental pancreatic cancer induced by dimethylbenzanthracene in mice. Cancer Science. 2007;**98**(2):155-162. DOI: 10.1111/j.1349-7006.2006.00369.x

[13] Clemons M, Goss P. Estrogen and the risk of breast cancer. The New England Journal of Medicine. 2001;**344**(4):276-285. DOI: 10.1056/NEJM200101253440407

[14] Benakanakere I, Besch-Williford C, Carroll CE, Hyder SM. Synthetic progestins differentially promote or prevent DMBA-induced mammary tumors in Sprague-dawley rats. Cancer Prevention Research (Philadelphia, Pa.). 2010;**3**(9):1157-1167. DOI: 10.1158/1940-6207.CAPR-10-0064

[15] Ohi Y, Yoshida H. Influence of estrogen and progesterone on the induction of mammary carcinomas by 7,12-dimethylbenz (a) anthracene in ovariectomized rats. Virchows Archiv. B, Cell Pathology Including Molecular Pathology. 1992;**62**(6):365-370. DOI: 10.1007/BF02899705

[16] Lakhani S, Ellis I, Schnitt S, et al. WHO Classification of Tumours of the Breast. 4th ed. Lyon: IARC Press; 2012

[17] Vuong D, Simpson PT, Green B, Cummings MC, Lakhani SR. Molecular classification of breast cancer. Virchows Archiv. 2014;**465**(1):1-14. DOI: 10.1007/s00428-014-1593-7

[18] Alvarado A, Lopes AC, Faustino-Rocha AI, Cabrita MS, Ferreira R, Oliveira PA, et al. Animal and in vitro model prognostic factors in MNU and DMBA-induced mammary tumors in female rats. Pathology, Research and Practice. 2017;**213**(5):441-446. DOI: 10.1016/j.prp.2017.02.014

[19] Masood S. Breast cancer subtypes: Morphologic and biologic characterization. Womens Health (Lond). 2016;**12**(1):103-119. DOI: 10.2217/whe.15.99

[20] Klopfleisch R, Euler H, Sarli G, Pinho SS, Gärtner F, Gruber AD. Molecular carcinogenesis of canine mammary tumors: News from an old disease. Veterinary Pathology. 2011;**48**(1):98-116. DOI: 10.1177/0300985810390826

Chapter 4

Neurodegeneracy

Safiya Tazeen and Mohammed Ibrahim

Abstract

Despite its vulnerability to neurodegenerative diseases, the neuromuscular junction has developed powerful ways to withstand injury and regenerate. Individuals with neurodegenerative diseases have a shorter life expectancy. Most existing treatments for neurodegenerative diseases only address symptoms. In order to limit the harmful effects, it is important to develop successful therapies to setback the symptoms of these debilitating diseases. Though some neurodegenerative disorders are fatal, most lead to health complications that are associated with high mortality rates. Although this difference might be a matter of semantics, we consider it significant, not only for managing the patient but also for our understanding of the actual consequences of the neurodegenerative process.

Keywords: neuron, oxidative stress, dementia, glial cells, astrocytes

1. Introduction

Neurodegeneration describes a complex and serious medical condition, which principally affects the neurons. Such a situation leads to disorders of the central nervous system.

Degenerative nerve affects various body activities such as balance, movement, talking, heart functioning, breathing, mood swing, poor coordination, seizure, confusion, and altered levels of consciousness in other words it affects day-to-day life. The basis of such dysfunction can be quite varied.

Neurological disorders can influence the entire neurologic pathway or a single neuron. Even a little disturbance to a neuron's structural pathway can result in dysfunction.

Neurological disorders can result from a number of sources that includes lifestyle, nutrition, environmental influences, physical injuries, infections including defective protein degradation and aggregation, free radical formation, oxidative stress and exposure to metal toxicity and pesticides.

The central nervous system consists of two types of cells, neurons and glial cells. Electrical impulses are not produced by glial cells, they are the supporting cells of neurons. These glial cells are superior to neurons in their function and cellular diversity. Glial cells including microglia, oligodendrocytes, and astrocytes, can regulate neuronal action.

Typically, the development of neurodegeneration initiates in the subcortical region as the disease progresses and extends to cortical regions [1]. Primary loss of neurons varies with the disease like striatal and cortical regions in HD, striatal regions in PD, spinal motor neurons and cortical regions in ALS, and hippocampal and cortical regions in AD [2–4].

Neurodegenerative diseases consider sharing a common pathogenic mechanism relating to aggregation and deposition of misfolded proteins, leading to unavoidable progressive worsening of the central nervous system. Misfolded proteins may create the most trouble as they form protofibrils. A number of methods have been described. In a few cases, these are particularly related to the type of protein, but in many other cases, they are nonspecific mechanisms shared by every misfolded protein disease. For a normal function, a protein must be properly synthesised and folded into its normal three-dimensional configuration. Nascent proteins are served in folding by molecular chaperones. Improperly folded proteins either damaged or otherwise beyond their functional lives are degraded by a ubiquitin-dependent proteasome protein degradation system.

In this system initially, the proteins are labelled for degradation by attachment of a polyubiquitin chain. Protein fragments and polyubiquitin are the end products of proteasome action. This polyubiquitin is then degraded and also recycled to the cellular ubiquitin pool, this process required enzymatic action by ubiquitin carboxy-terminal hydrolase 1.

The subject of strong investigation is the cascade of pathogenic actions linking abnormal protein aggregation to cell death. Even though aggregates are the most striking physical change in surviving cells, the actual function of the aggregate remains a mystery. Mostly it is believed that the formation of aggregates may be a protective mechanism sequestering the wayward protein from vulnerable cell procedure.

There is an emerging proof that performed fibrils generated from the full length and truncated recombinant α-synuclein enter neurons, most likely by endocytosis, and act as "seeds" that stimulate the employment of soluble endogenous α-synuclein into soluble inclusions, resulting in progressive prion-like extend of neurodegeneration. The mutant protein may not be able to carry out a vital function or may obstruct the function of the wild-type protein. Mutant proteins may operate the apoptotic cascade. They may impede intracellular transport or other vital activities. They may restrain the activity of the proteasome, increasing protein aggregation. They may get in the way of mitochondrial function, making cells more exposed to excitotoxicity. Lysosomes play an essential role in ubiquitin–proteasome system in degrading intracellular proteins. When the function of the ubiquitin-proteasome system is not enough to clear the accumulating cellular protein, then the autophagy-lysosome pathway turns into the other main direction for the degradation of misfolded proteins as well as unwell mitochondria. For maintaining cellular health mitophagy is a highly recognised mechanism.

With the ageing of the population, the occurrence of neurodegeneration is escalating spectacularly in the absence of either effective therapeutic involvement or a clear understanding of the separate pathophysiology of neurodegenerative disease states.

Currently, a few hundred neurodegenerative diseases have been estimated and among these, many appear to overlap with one another pathologically and clinically, leaving their practical categorisation challenging to a certain extent. In diseases the issue is further complicated by multisystem atrophy where quite a lot of areas of the brain are affected, different combinations of lesions can give different clinical pictures. Moreover, the same neurodegenerative processes, in particular at the beginning, can affect different areas of the brain, making a known given disease appear very different from a symptomatic standpoint. In spite of these difficulties, the most popular classification of neurodegenerative disorders is still o the bases of the predominant clinical feature or the topography of the predominant lesion, or frequently on a combination of both.

2. Sleep and neurodegeneration

Dementia is described by a progressive decline of reminiscence and cognition followed by language dysfunction, depression, hallucinations, other psychotic features, and sleep disturbance. In advanced phases, the patient turns out to be mute, bedridden and incontinent. The chief sleep disturbances in dementing illness include hypersomnia, insomnia, extreme nocturnal motor action, circadian sleep/wake rhythm disorders, respiratory dysrhythmias and "sundowning".

Synthesis of new extracellular matrix protein takes place in reactive astrocytes in the areas of neural degeneration that provide boundaries to segregate damaged axons from healthy axons, prevent hematogenous cells from invading the offended neural tissues, affect the survival of remaining axons, and prevent axonal regrowth.

3. Classification and molecular characteristics of neurotraumatic disease

Neurodegeneration is a complex multifactorial progression that causes neuronal death in the brain and spinal cord, resulting in brain and spinal cord injury and dysfunction. Neurodegeneration along with axonal transport shortage, oxidative stress, protein oligomerization, aggregation, mitochondrial dysfunction, calcium deregulation, DNA damage, irregular neuron-glial interactions, neuroinflammation and abnormal RNA processing.

Neurodegeneration happens in neurotraumatic, neurodegenerative, and neuropsychiatric diseases. These diseases occur due to neurochemical, structural and electrophysiological aberrations in the brain, spinal cord, and nerve bringing out muscle weakness, paralysis, seizures, uncertainty, poor coordination and soreness. Neurodegenerative diseases entail the accretion of misfolded proteins and the beginning of neurodegenerative diseases, some nutrients, oxygen and ATP are accessible to the neurons, ion homeostasis is maintained to a limited point, and neurodegeneration takes a longer time to die.

Neuropsychiatric disorders are schizophrenia, depression, autism, bipolar effective disorders, attention-deficit disorder, tardive dyskinesia, and chronic fatigue syndrome.

Neurodegeneration encircles multiple molecular ways and a complex interplay between different regulatory factors together with the epigenetic mechanism. Although traditional drugs target various etiological mechanisms in separation, one should concentrate on drugs which have multiple therapeutic objectives and can be given either as monotherapy or as adjunctive drugs for effective results.

4. Neurodegeneration with Brain Iron Accumulation (NBIA)

The latest molecular studies revealed the existence of inherited neurodegenerative disorders, termed "neurodegeneration with brain iron accumulation" (NBIA), owing to genetic faults associated with iron metabolism. NBIA is a heterogeneous set of disorders that comprises "Pantothenate Kinase-Associated Neurodegeneration" (PKAN), infantile neuroaxonal defect, and neuroferritinopathy. Together, these disorders share similarities in extrapyramidal neurodegeneration and focal Fe accumulation, frequently in the basal ganglia and further brain regions including the thalamus, SN, cerebellar dentate nucleus and red nucleus. Symptoms comprise disablement in movement and cognition. NBIA consists of a series of disorders, a few caused by a mutation in a well-distinguished metalloprotein.

Along with iron accumulation, lipid peroxidation and mitochondrial damage are involved in both NBIA and ferroptosis, signifying the role of ferroptosis in the development of neurodegenerative diseases.

The general neurodegenerative diseases following TBI (Traumatic Brain Injury) resemble Parkinson's disease (PD) and Alzheimer's disease (AD) too share identical characteristics with ferroptosis, such as overload iron and lipid peroxidation.

Unique with iron excess syndromes, aceruloplasminemia (iron accumulation in the brain and other organs) involves together systemic and brain iron metabolism. A noticeable build-up of iron in the affected parenchymal tissues, namely the liver, pancreas, thyroid, and heart, the outcome in cardiac failure and hypothyroidism. The systemic tissues with access to iron are the reason for disrupted tissue iron release, followed by incorporation into circulating transferrin.

5. Neurological disorders

There are numerous distinguished neurological disorders, and a number of them are common, but many are rare. They may be evaluated by neurological assessment, studied and treated by the expertise of neuropsychology. Neurological disorders can be classified according to the primary affected area because the primary cause is most important and the wide division is between the central nervous system and peripheral nervous system disorders. Neurological disorders can influence the whole neurological pathway or a neuron alone. Even a little trouble with a neuron's structural pathways can consequence in dysfunction.

There are numerous mechanisms of pathogenesis involved in the progress of neurodegenerative disorders. Internal and external stressors can cause activation of neuroglial cells which involves the disturbance of normal nervous functions and triggers the process of apoptosis in the neuronal cells. A small portion of neurodegenerative diseases are due to the mutation of disease-related genes, but the majority of them are sporadic where environmental issues and ageing plays a predominant role. Disturbance of cellular function from ageing- stimulates the accumulation of neuronal stressors resulting in cell death. Though, there is somewhat little neuronal loss in normal ageing, while cell death is a general characteristic of neurodegenerative diseases.

In the homeostatic regulation of physiological and pathological functions, redox balance plays an important role. When surplus free radicals cannot be eradicated, the accumulation stimulates and leads to "oxidative stress". The reactive oxygen species (ROS) accumulation can cause damage to mitochondrial DNA, agitating the reliability of the energy cycle, which is necessary for neurological growth and function.

Neuronal tissue inflammation happens due to the accumulation of ROS, which encourages the synthesis of cytokines and other inflammatory mediators by triggering the inflammation pathway.

Antioxidant therapy represents an assuring possibility for the treatment of neurological diseases. Even though the difficulty and inconsistency of redox biology have mostly avoided the analysis of the mechanisms of and therapeutic approaches for neurological disease.

The lack of early diagnosis and cure for neurodegenerative diseases is always to be a huge confront for society.

6. Neurodegenerative disorders

6.1 Agnosia

In this disorder the ability to identify objects, persons, sound, shapes or smells are lost while the specific sense is neither defective nor is there any considerable memory loss. Usually, it is correlated with brain injury or neurological illness, especially after damage to the right parietal lobe.

6.2 Alexander disease

It is a gradually progressing and mortal neurodegenerative disease. It is an atypical disorder which results from a genetic mutation and generally has an effect on infants and children, causing developmental obstacles and changes once physical characteristics.

6.3 Alpers disease

A rare degenerative disease of the brain connecting the grey matter. It is described by the acute initiation of severe convulsions that lead to a speedy intellectual and bodily breakdown. Other features are deafness, myoclonus, blindness, choreo-athetosis, spasticity, cerebellar ataxia, growth delay, plus terminal decortications. Noticeable in early childhood and generally causes death within a month.

6.4 Alzheimer's disease

The disease of the brain progresses slowly and is characterised by the devastation of memory and ultimately disturbance in planning, language, reasoning and perception.

6.5 Apraxia

This neurological disorder is described by the loss of ability to perform learned determined movements, even though having the desire to perform the physical activities. It is a disorder of motor planning which may be obtained or developmental, but it is may not be caused by sensory loss, in coordination.

6.6 Batten disease

It begins in childhood, a rare, deadly, autosomal recessive neurodegenerative disorder. It is also known as "Spielmeyer-Vogt-Sjogren-Batten" disease, it is one of the most common forms of disorders called NCLs (neuronal ceroid lipofuscinosis).

6.7 Benign essential blepharospasm

It is a progressive neurological disorder differentiated by involuntary muscle contractions and spasms of the eyelid muscles.

6.8 Canavan disease

It is one of the most general cerebral degenerative diseases of infancy, is a gene-linked, neurological birth disorder where the white matter of the brain degenerates into spongy tissue puzzled with microscopic fluid that filled the spaces. This disease is known as leukodystrophy a group of genetic disorders, which cause faulty development or growth of myelin sheath, the fatty covering that work as an insulator around nerve fibres in the brain. Canavan disease is caused by a mutation in the gene used for an enzyme called aspartoacylase.

6.9 Cerebral beriberi

Also known as "Wernicke's Encephalopathy" is a degenerative brain disorder due to the lack of Vit B1(thiamin). It may be the result of alcohol abuse, prolonged vomiting, eating disorders, and dietary deficiencies.

6.10 Corticobasal degeneration

A continuous neurological disorder described by nerve cell loss and shrinkage of multiple regions of the brain including the cerebral cortex and the basal ganglia, this progress gradually and initial symptoms begin around age 60.

6.11 Dementia

Also called "Semantic Frontotemporal Dementia" (FTD) shows a clinical syndrome linked with the shrinking of the frontal and temporal anterior lobes of the brain.

6.12 Hallervorden Spatz disease

Also Known as "Neurodegeneration with Brain Iron Accumulation" (NBIA) is an exceptional, inherited, neurological movement disorder describe by progressive degeneration of the nervous system.

6.13 Huntington's disease

It is an inherited neurodegenerative disorder of the central nervous system, deteriorating and always fatal, this can cause progressive degeneration of cells in the brain, gradually weakening an individual's ability to think, talk, walk and reason.

6.14 Lou Gehrig's disease

Also known as "Amyotrophic Lateral Sclerosis" (ALS), a quickly progressive, constantly fatal neurological disease that attacks the neurons responsible for controlling voluntary muscle. In ALS the upper and lower motor neurons degenerate and stopping to send messages to muscles.

6.15 Mitochondrial myopathies

A group of neuromuscular diseases caused due to damage to the mitochondria, the energy-producing structures called the "powerhouse of the cell". Neurons in the brain and muscles need a great deal of energy, this appears to be damaged when mitochondrial dysfunction occurs.

6.16 Neuronal Ceriod lipofuscinosis

This is the result of excessive accumulation of lipopigments in the body tissues. In general, it is the name for a family of at least eight genetically separate neurodegenerative disorders.

6.17 Neuronal migration disorders

These are the group of birth defects originating from the atypical migration of neurons in the developing brain and nervous system.

6.18 Olivopontocerebellar atrophy

The term (OPCA) is used to describe neurological degeneration in the cerebellum, pontine nuclei, and inferior olive. OPCA can also originate in the brains of an individual with prion disorders and inherited metabolic diseases. The distinctive regions of the damaged brain by OPCA can be seen by imaging the brain using CT scan or MRI studies.

6.19 O'Sullivan-McLeod syndrome

Also known as "Monomelic Amyotrophy" (MMA) and is illustrated by progressive degeneration and loss of motor neurons, the nerve cells of the brain and spinal cord, responsible for controlling voluntary muscles.

6.20 Paraneoplastic syndromes

It is a collection of rare degenerative disorders that are generated by a person's immune system response to a neoplasm. It is believed to cause when cancer-fighting antibodies by mistake hit normal cells in the nervous system.

6.21 Pelizaeus-Merzbacher disease

It is a group of a gene linked to rare progressive, degenerative central nervous system disorders where motor skills, coordination and intellectual function deteriorate.

6.22 Prion disease

It is also known as "Transmissible Spongiform Encephalopathies" (TSEs), a rare group of degenerative brain disorders describe by minute holes that cause the brain a "spongy" appearance.

6.23 Sandhoff disease

It is caused due to the deficiency of the enzyme beta-hexosaminidase, which is the result of the accumulation of certain fats in the brain and other organs of the body. It is a rare, genetic disorder resulting in a progressive decline of the central nervous system.

6.24 Shy-Drager syndrome

It is a neurological disorder also known as multiple system atrophy with orthostatic hypotension causes dizziness and fainting. Doctors classify the disorder into 3 types

- Parkinsonian type includes symptoms of Parkinson's disease.
- Cerebellar type causes problems with coordination and speech.
- The combined type includes symptoms of both parkinsonism and cerebellar failure.

It is a progressive disorder of the central and autonomic nervous systems were problems with urinary incontinence, weakness double vision, constipation and decreased sweating.

6.25 Tabes dorsalis

It is a slow degeneration of the nerve cells and nerve fibres that transmit sensory information to the brain. These nerves are in the dorsal columns of the spinal cord and carry out a signal which helps to maintain an individual's sense of position.

7. Recent progress in preventing neurodegenerative diseases

It is known that neurological disorder which includes Alzheimer's disease (AD), Multiple sclerosis (MS), Parkinson's disease (PD), Huntington's disease (HD), and Amyotrophic lateral sclerosis (ALS) that noticeable in millions of people throughout the world every year. The common feature of these disorders is neuronal loss and the outcome is locomotor difficulties, cognitive defects, and chronic deterioration in memory.

Hence the researchers are following a collaborative approach to preserving the function and groups of neural tissues before the damage. This neuroprotective approach concentrates on the improvement in strategies that prevent most neuronal death.

8. Prevention of self-directed neurodegeneration

To maintain and restore physiological homeostasis cell has a variety of self-repair mechanism. Whenever a cell loses the capacity to overcome the damage, intracellular homeostasis falls and stimulates a series of cell death events takes place. Research over a few years and studies have shown that apoptotic cell death is not the only pathway directing the loss in these disorders. Among them, poly (ADP-ribose)

(PAR)-dependent cell death has been started as being responsible for neuronal loss in various neurological disorders, comprising AD, ALS, HD, and PD. Oxidative stress injured DNA, resulting in PAR1 activation due to excessive accumulation of intracellular PARP1 [5]. Parthanatos is the result of numerous cellular processes, consisting release of apoptosis-inducing factor (AIF) from mitochondria, overactivation and macrophage migration inhibitory factor (MIF) and co-translocation of AIF into the nucleus, directing to DNA fragmentation and cell death [6, 7].

Overactivation of PARP1 and PAR accumulation have been noticed in the brains of AD patients [8, 9]. Studies have revealed that neurons are guarded by PARP1 inhibition, which means that PARP1 inhibition may have therapeutic importance for the treatment of AD.

Modern discoveries in the PD model show more direct facts that in pathologic α-synuclein neurodegeneration, parthanatos is the most important cell death pathway. In this PAR is the main mediator, encouraging α-synuclein toxicity and fibril conducting, exacerbating neurotoxicity in a feed-forward loop [10]. Oral administration of PARP1 inhibitor and genetic reduction of PARP1 stopped neurodegeneration and progresses motor capability in both genetic and sporadic models of PD [10, 11]. Moreover, increased PAR levels in the cerebral spinal fluid and brains of patients with PD [10], recommend that PARP1 might be a theragnostic biomarker and a disease-modifying therapeutic goal in PD [12]. Elongated polyglutamine (poly Q) is responsible for Huntington (htt) protein aggregation along with neuronal inclusions and toxicity in HD [13].

Enhanced PAR levels and dysregulation of PARP1 activation contribute to the pathogenesis of several neurodegenerative diseases by promoting parthanatos and protein aggregation. Therefore, a neuroprotective course of action intended to reduce PARP1 activation may have therapeutic potential in those disorders. Several well-described PARP inhibitors are in experimental use and yet to be tested for use in neurodegenerative disorders [14]. Thus these can be regarded as a neuroprotective treatment for neurological disorders.

9. Impede of non-cell-autonomous neurodegeneration

In neuronal support, glial cells play a key role in maintaining homeostasis, neurogenesis and nutrient transportation in healthy brains, [15]. Notably, an emerging research body has shown that dysfunctional non-neuronal cells such as astrocytes and microglia straight supply to neurodegeneration and cell death (Thus called non-cell autonomous neurodegeneration) in several neurodegenerative disorders.

Microglia are the inhabitant macrophages and primary immune cells in the brain. Hence they play a significant role in neuronal disease. In the post-mortem of AD brains, reactive microglia are present and have been shown to encourage synaptic drop and neuroinflammation [16, 17]. In the glial cells many PD-related genes, incorporating α-synuclein, PINK1, and parkin, are expressed. During PD pathogenesis mutated gene products are engaged in microglial dysfunction.

In review, microglia is believed to have both useful and harmful functions in neurodegenerative diseases. Therefore, the introduction of subsequent prevention of neurotoxic microglia signature and DAM (disease-associated microglia) or homeostatic microglia signature could be assuring therapeutic approaches for neuroprotection in neurodegenerative diseases, but the elements allied with heterogenous microglial phenotype will require to be defined in further detail.

The most abundant population of glial cells in the CNS is the astrocytes which carry out a broad range of homeostatic functions. So it is not surprising that the loss of the usual normal astrocyte role is engaged in the pathogenesis of neurodegenerative diseases. According to a 2017 investigation, activated microglia induce the formation of neurotoxic reactive astrocytes by releasing interleukin 1α (IL-1α), tumour necrosis factor α (TNF-α), and C1q [18]. In the post-mortem of the human brain, neurodegenerative diseases like AD, PD, ALS, and HD reactive astrocytes were found [18].

Currently, though, it has been observed that the phenotype variety of astrocytes is noticed in brains with neurodegenerative diseases and widens beyond the A1 and A2 phenotypes [19–24]. Hence further research is required to know more about the molecular mechanisms of reactive astrocytes and their particular role within different neurodegenerative pathologies, specifically how the neurotoxic signals interchange and are shared across multiple neurodegenerative conditions.

10. Conclusion

There is a number of factors which cause neurodegenerative diseases such as neuronal cell death, genetic mutations, protein aggregation, flawed protein recycling, mitochondrial dysfunction, and innate immune responses due to glial cell activation. Hence neuroprotection can be achieved from cell-autonomous neurodegeneration directly by attacking their neighbouring cells. Thus, to prevent or slow neurodegeneration a multifaceted approach attacking both cell-autonomous and non-cell-autonomous mechanisms may be required.

To understand neurodegeneration, the molecular mechanism is an important footstep in the development of novel neuroprotective therapies. Due to remarkable efforts, these therapies have developed beyond the lab to the clinical testing stage. Thus, further research in the neurodegenerative pathways and the development and identification of neuroprotective agents are required to build up promising disease-modifying therapeutic approaches for the management, handling, and treatment of the neurodegenerative diseases.

Author details

Safiya Tazeen* and Mohammed Ibrahim
KBN University, Gulbarga, India

*Address all correspondence to: tazeenchishti@gmail.com

References

[1] Zhou J, Gennatas ED, Kramer JH, Miller BL, Seeley WW. Predicting regional neurodegeneration from the healthy brain functional connectome. Neuron. 2012;**73**:1216-1227

[2] Ilieva H, Polymenidou M, Cleveland DW. Non–cell autonomous toxicity in neurodegenerative disorders: ALS and beyond. The Journal of Cell Biology. 2009;**187**:761-772

[3] Kiaei M. New hopes and challenges for treatment of neurodegenerative disorders: Great opportunities for young neuroscientists. Basic Clinical Neuroscience. 2013;**4**:3-4

[4] Marambaud P, Dreses-Werringloer U, Vingtdeux V. Calcium signaling in neurodegeneration. Molecular Neurodegeneration. 2009;**4**:20

[5] Park H, Kam TI, Dawson TM, et al. Poly (ADP-ribose) (PAR)-dependent cell death in neurodegenerative diseases. International Review of Cell and Molecular Biology. 2020a;**2020**(353):1-29

[6] Wang Y, Kim NS, Haince JF, et al. Poly (ADP-ribose) (PAR) binding to apoptosis-inducing factor is critical for PAR polymerase-1-dependent cell death (parthanatos). Science Signaling. 2011;**4**(167)

[7] Wang Y, Kim NS, Li X, et al. Calpain activation is not required for AIF translocation in PARP-1-dependent cell death (parthanatos). Journal of Neurochemistry. 2009;**110**(2):687-696

[8] Love S, Barber R, Wilcock GK. Increased poly(ADP-ribosyl)ation of nuclear proteins in Alzheimer's disease. Brain. 1999;**122**(Pt 2):247-253

[9] Martire S, Fuso A, Rotili D, et al. PARP-1 modulates amyloid beta peptide-induced neuronal damage. PLoS One. 2013;**8**(9):e72169

[10] Kam TI, Mao X, Park H, et al. Poly(ADP-ribose) drives pathologic α-synuclein neurodegeneration in Parkinson's disease. Science. 2018;**362**(6414):eaat8407

[11] Mao K, Chen J, Yu H, et al. Poly (ADP-ribose) polymerase 1 inhibition prevents neurodegeneration and promotes α-synuclein degeneration via transcription factor EB-dependent autophagy in mutant α-synucleinA53T model of Parkinson's disease. Aging Cell. 2020;**19**(6)

[12] Olsen AL, Feany MB. PARP inhibitors and Parkinson's disease. The New England Journal of Medicine. 2019;**380**(5):492-494

[13] Williams AJ, Paulson HL. Polyglutamine neurodegeneration: Protein misfolding revisited. Trends in Neurosciences. 2008;**31**(10):521-528

[14] Berger NA, Besson VC, Boulares AH, et al. Opportunities for the repurposing of PARP inhibitors for the therapy of non-oncological diseases. British Journal of Pharmacology. 2018;**175**(2): 192-222

[15] Wang G, Zhou Y, Wang Y, et al. Age-associated dopaminergic neuron loss and midbrain glia cell phenotypic polarization. Neuroscience. 2019;**415**:89-96

[16] Rajendran L, Paolicelli RC. Microglia-mediated synapse loss in Alzheimer's disease. The Journal of Neuroscience. 2018;**38**(12):2911-2919

[17] Van der Kant R, Goldstein LSB, Ossenkoppele R. Amyloid-β-independent regulators of tau pathology in Alzheimer disease. Nature Reviews. Neuroscience. 2020;**21**(1):21-35

[18] Liddelow SA, Guttenplan KA, Clarke LE, et al. Neurotoxic reactive astrocytes are induced by activated microglia. Nature. 2017;**541**(7638):481-487

[19] Al-Dalahmah O, Sosunov AA, Shaik A, et al. Single-nucleus RNA-seq identifies Huntington disease astrocyte states. Acta Neuropathologica Communications. 2020;**8**(1):19

[20] Das S, Li Z, Noori A, et al. Meta-analysis of mouse transcriptomic studies supports a context-dependent astrocyte reaction in acute CNS injury versus neurodegeneration. Journal of Neuroinflammation. 2020, 2020;**17**(1):227

[21] Diaz-Castro B, Gangwani MR, Yu X, et al. Astrocyte molecular signatures in Huntington's disease. Science Translational Medicine. 2019;**11**(514):eaaw8546

[22] Grubman A, Chew G, Ouyang JF, et al. A single-cell atlas of entorhinal cortex from individuals with Alzheimer's disease reveals cell-type-specific gene expression regulation. Nature Neuroscience. 2019;**22**(12):2087-2097

[23] Wheeler MA, Clark IC, Tjon EC, et al. MAFG-driven astrocytes promote CNS inflammation. Nature. 2020;**578**(7796):593-599

[24] Zhou Y, Song WM, Andhey PS, et al. Human and mouse single-nucleus transcriptomics reveal TREM2-dependent and TREM2-independent cellular responses in Alzheimer's disease. Nature Medicine. 2020;**26**(1):131-142

Chapter 5

Application of New Nanostructured Materials in Furcation Defects Therapy

Marijana Popović Bajić, Violeta Petrović, Vanja Opačić Galić, Smiljana Paraš, Vukoman Jokanović and Slavoljub Živković

Abstract

The potential use of calcium phosphate cements in endodontic therapy is an active area of research. Hydroxyapatite is one of the most commonly used calcium phosphate materials in medicine and dentistry. Biocompatibility of hydroxyapatite is closely related to its chemical composition, similar to dental and bony tissues. Recent studies have focused on new and modified formulations of calcium-phosphate-based biomaterials with improved mechanical and maintained favorable biological properties. Recently, two non-commercial new nanomaterials based on calcium silicates and hydroxyapatite have been synthesized. One is a calcium silicate system of tricalcium and dicalcium silicates (CS), and the other one is a mixture of the calcium silicate system and hydroxyapatite (HA-CS). Both CS and HA-CS are nanostructural materials. Particle size affects cement hydration and consequently setting time and final quality of the cement. Fast setting is a clear clinical advantage while cement composition and internal nanostructure are expected to provide biological behavior in vital tissues. The problem with furcation perforation repair is still not agreed upon as no currently available materials meet all the requirements of an ideal repair material as defined in the literature. Therefore, this study aimed to compare the tissue reaction of two new repair materials for furcation perforations.

Keywords: calcium silicate cement, hydroxyapatite, nanotechnology, furcation defects, nanostructured materials

1. Introduction

Root perforations represent communication between the root canal system of the tooth and the outer surface of the tooth root. Most often, they arise as a result of pathological processes, such as deep caries or resorption, and are revealed by a detailed clinical examination or X-ray analysis. However, most perforations occur mechanically, due to iatrogenic factors (during the opening of the access cavity, finding the entrance to the canals, mechanical processing of the root canal, or during the preparation phase for an intracanal post) [1–4]. The resulting iatrogenic perforations affect the success of endodontic therapy and the long-term prognosis of the tooth. Root perforations leading to failure of endodontic treatment account for approximately 10% of all failures [5]. Errors during endodontic therapy can occur at any stage of the work. Predisposing factors for the occurrence of perforations are the presence of denticles, calcification, obliterated canals, internal resorptions, inability to identify canal orifices, extensive caries, inclined or rotated teeth, and presence of canal posts [1–4]. Root perforation is a serious complication that requires rapid diagnosis, and timely and adequate therapy. Root perforations often lead to an inflammatory response and destruction of periodontal tissue and alveolar bone. The proliferation of granulomatous tissue, the proliferation of the epithelium, the formation of an endoperiodontal lesion and finally the loss of teeth can occur depending on the size of the perforation, its localization, and the intensity of the chronic inflammatory reaction [1, 6, 7].

Perforations of single-rooted teeth have a better prognosis than perforations of multi-rooted teeth. Perforations in the furcation area of multi-rooted teeth are a special problem. Iatrogenic perforations in the area of the furcation occur in approximately 2–12% of endodontically treated teeth and can have serious consequences on the outcome of endodontic therapy, but also on the preservation of the tooth itself [1, 8]. This perforation is an open door for bacteria to enter, either from the root canal or from the periodontal tissue, which causes an intense inflammatory response. The consequences of the inflammatory reaction can be bone resorption, growth of the gingival epithelium, and the appearance of a fistula, which further worsens the prognosis of the tooth [1].

Factors that determine the prognosis of a tooth with a perforation include the size and localization of the defect, the time elapsed from the diagnosis to the closure of the perforation, the duration of the contamination, the physical and chemical properties of the material used for its repair, or its sealing capabilities [9, 10]. The prognosis would be relatively good if the perforation was quickly detected and closed with a biocompatible material [11, 12]. There are now various biocompatible materials on the market that are used to close perforations in order to reduce the inflammatory reaction in the surrounding tissues [13–15]. The ideal material for closing these perforations should be non-toxic, non-resorbable, radiopaque, bactericidal, or bacteriostatic, and should provide a hermetic seal and prevent microleakage [16, 17].

In the literature, calcium silicate-based materials are most often used for such clinical situations. They are used in direct pulp capping procedures, closure of the root apex in apex surgery, therapy of root perforations, pulpotomy, and apexification [18, 19]. Biocompatibility, bioactivity, and sealing ability of calcium silicate cement have been proven in many studies due to their potential for dentin, cementum, bone, and periodontal ligament regeneration [18, 19]. The good biological properties of calcium-silicate cement are associated with calcium hydroxide, which is released during the bonding of the material and stimulates the proliferation and differentiation of various cells for tissue regeneration [20].

Mineral trioxide aggregate (MTA) was introduced in endodontics in 1990, as a new material with the property of closing the communication between the tooth and the outer surface of the root [18, 19]. *In vitro* and *in vivo* studies have shown that MTA has significant sealing ability and marginal adaptation [18, 19]. This material has a long initial setting time (3 h), as a result of its chemical composition and hygroscopic nature, and it also contains traces of heavy metals [21]. MTA contains bismuth oxide as an X-ray contrast agent, which interferes with cement hydration processes [22] and can react with dentin collagen, leading to tooth discoloration [23]. Newer generations of MTA cement have a slightly shorter initial setting time, as a result of changes in chemical composition, and contain non-toxic radiocontrast agents such as zirconium oxide [24]. The main disadvantages of MTA are the long setting time and difficult handling of this material, despite its optimal sealing ability and other advantages [25].

Despite its biocompatibility and bioconductivity, hydroxyapatite has not found its place in endodontic therapy, mainly due to inadequate mechanical properties. In order to improve the mechanical properties and bioactivity of hydroxyapatite, it was added to calcium silicate cements [26].

Technological progress and the influence of nanotechnology in the field of biomedical research have led to the emergence of new nanostructured materials. This new field of science deals with controlling matter, energy and/or information at the atomic and molecular level and enables the synthesis of new materials that are increasingly similar to natural biomolecular structures [27].

Nanomedicine is a branch of medicine that is based on the medical application of nanotechnologies, through the application of nanomaterials, nanoelectronic biosensors, and molecular nanotechnology [27, 28]. The very size of nanomaterial particles (< 100 nm), which is similar to the size of biological molecules and structures (proteins 5 nm, organelles 100–200 nm), points to the possible application of nanomaterials in *in vivo* and *in vitro* biomedical research [29]. Nanomedicines made from nanomaterials and nanoparticles (compared to drugs made from the same materials in a classical way) have up to ten times greater interactive surface, which unequivocally indicates a possible improvement in the pharmacokinetic and pharmacodynamic properties of the drug. Chen (2012) points out that the bioactivity, biocompatibility, stability, and mechanical properties of nanomaterials are determined by their composition, structure, morphology, and crystal size, as well as the method of synthesis [30].

Nanomaterials have revolutionized medicine and are increasingly being used in this field. These materials have the ability to mimic the surface properties of natural tissues, are highly cytocompatible and biocompatible, and therefore show excellent properties for use in tissue engineering and regenerative medicine [27]. The pronounced activity of nanoparticles improves the hydration of nanostructured calcium silicate cement, improving their hardening and bonding, as well as their physical and chemical properties [31]. However, there are concerns about the biological behavior of these materials, as nanoparticles usually deposit in mitochondria, causing structural damage to cells. Commercial nanostructured calcium silicate cement with hydroxyapatite (BioAggregate, Innovative bioceramics, Vancouver, BC, Canada) shows similar toxicity in cell cultures, but lower systemic toxicity compared to commercial MTA, which was related to differences in the content of heavy metals and differences in production [32].

Two new experimental nanostructured cements were recently developed at the Institute of Nuclear Sciences "Vinča" according to the recipe of V. Jokanović and associates. The goal was to synthesize materials with good biological properties, short bonding time, and without heavy metals and bismuth oxide. The first cement (CS) was based on dicalcium and tricalcium silicate, and the second (HA-CS) was a mixture of hydroxyapatite with CS, in a ratio of 2:1. CS was synthesized using a hydrothermal sol-gel methodology and self-propagating combustion waves [33]. Hydroxyapatite was synthesized by the hydrothermal method. Both materials contain barium sulfate as an X-ray contrast agent. The setting time of CS and HA-CS is 10 minutes and 15 minutes. *In vitro* testing of CS and HA-CS showed no genotoxic effects on human cells [34]. Their biocompatibility was confirmed in studies where these materials were applied in subcutaneous tissue in rats or as direct pulp capping material in rabbits [35, 36].

Examination of the cytotoxicity of these materials on cell culture of fibroblasts and MRC-5 cells showed better results in comparison with MTA [37].

Calcium silicate hydrate gel (CSH) and calcium hydroxide, the main soluble fraction of cement that dissolves into Ca^{2+} and OH^- ions, are formed by the hydration of calcium silicate materials. The reaction of released calcium with phosphates from tissue fluids represents the physicochemical basis of the bioactivity of calcium silicate materials [38]. It was established that the formation of an apatite layer on the surface of the material is not only a consequence of the release of calcium, but also the formation of Si-OH groups on the surface of the cement, which acts as centers of apatite nucleation and precipitation. Consequently, the synergistic action of calcium silicate hydrate gel as an apatite nucleator and calcium from dissolved calcium hydroxide as a precipitation accelerator is responsible for the rapid precipitation of apatite. Additionally, the hydrophilic substrate facilitates the bond with the apatite layer due to the presence of OH- groups on the surface of the cement [39]. The formation of apatite on the surface of calcium silicate actually goes through several stages. Amorphous calcium phosphate first forms on the surface of the material and then transforms into apatite, which later matures into type B carbonate apatite, which represents the biological phase of hydroxyapatite of bone, cementum, and dentin.

Calcium silicate cements are superior to most of the endodontic materials known to date in terms of their biocompatibility, bioactivity, and sealing properties. The fact that they possess a strong inductive potential for the regeneration of damaged tissues has contributed to the fact that these cements are now considered the materials of choice for numerous clinical indications.

The improved physical properties of calcium silicate cements obtained by the application of nanotechnology in terms of lower degree of solubility, higher structural stability of the material, and shorter bonding time, as well as lower cytotoxicity and better biocompatibility of these materials [40, 41], are sufficient reasons for examining their application *in vivo* conditions. The chemical nature of the material and the method of synthesis should ensure satisfactory biological behavior of these materials in living tissues. Quality marginal sealing, that is, adequate marginal adaptation of the material, should prevent the flow of tissue fluids and consequent bacterial microleakage, which is a significant factor for the long-term success of endodontic treatment.

The aim of this study was to evaluate the inflammatory reactions of the periradicular tissue and the formation of calcified tissue after implantation of CS and HA-CS in the furcation defects of the teeth of Vietnamese pigs and in the root canals of the teeth of rabbits.

2. Experimental procedure

2.1 Application of CS and HA-CS in furcation defects of teeth of Vietnamese pigs

Experimental research was carried out at the Institute of Surgery of the Faculty of Veterinary Medicine, University of Belgrade, and at the Institute for Biological Research "Siniša Stanković," University of Belgrade.

Permission for experimental work with animals was obtained from the Ethics Committee of the Faculty of Veterinary Medicine and from the Ethics Committee of the Faculty of Dentistry (16/29), conducted according to international standards ISO10993-2 (Requirements for animal welfare) and ISO 7405.

Three Vietnamese pigs (*Sus scrofa* verus), both sexes, aged 24 months and with an average weight of 25 kg were the animal model in this experimental research. The protocol of the European Good Laboratory Practice (86/609/EEC), which implies the implementation of the main principles of asepsis and antisepsis, the realization of the experiment in the minimum necessary time without physical and mental pain of the animals (International Organization for Standardization, 1997), was respected during the work.

The animals were housed in the experimental animal facility at the Faculty of Veterinary Medicine, University of Belgrade, during the experiment. Each experimental animal was housed in an individual cage in a controlled environment with a controlled diet and daily professional care. The animals were provided with appropriate care, nutrition, hygienic conditions, and their health condition was checked 3 times a day.

The animals were deprived of food for 6 hours before the operation, and water for 3 hours before the operation, in order to rule out complications during the experiment. Premedication with atropine in a dose of 0.03–0.04 mg/kg by intramuscular injection was performed in all three animals, and after 15 minutes, the animals were put under general anesthesia by administering xylazine (2% Xylazin, Cp Pharma, Bergdorf, Germany) in a dose of 1.5–2 mg/kg and ketamine (Laboratorio Sanderso S.A., Santiago, Chile) at a dose of 20–25 mg/kg intramuscularly. The average duration of anesthesia was about 100 minutes.

The surgical procedure was performed under aseptic conditions and in a way that ensures minimal trauma. Each tooth was individually cleaned, dried, and disinfected (30% hydrogen and 70% ethanol). Access cavities were formed on the lower premolars with a round diamond bur. Coronary pulp tissue was removed with a sterile, carbide, round bur. Accidental perforation of the floor of the cavum dentis in the area of the furcation of the tooth was made with the same bur, 2 mm in diameter. The cavities were washed with 5 ml of physiological solution, and hemostasis was performed with sterile cotton balls, gently and without pressure. Freshly mixed experimental, nanostructured materials, CS, and HA-CS mixed with distilled water in a ratio of 2:1 were placed on the perforation [33]. All cavities were closed with glass ionomer cement (GC FUJI VIII, GC Corporation, Tokyo, Japan) as a definitive filling.

For the next 3 days, the animals were housed in the inpatient unit of the Institute of Surgery, under constant medical supervision with analgesic therapy (Butorphanol 0.1 mg/kg/tm/i.m. for 6 h). Appropriate care, nutrition, and hygienic conditions were provided to the animals during the observation period, and their health conditions were checked three times a day.

Experimental animals were sacrificed after 30 days, by intravenous injection of 10 ml of pentobarbiturate solution (100 mg/kg).

The mandible and maxilla were separated from the rest of the skull after the removal of the soft tissues, and the tissue was fixed in 10% formalin for 48 hours. The tissue for histological analysis was taken in the form of block sections, where each block consisted of an experimental tooth with the surrounding bone. The samples were decalcified in a decalcification solution: 8% HCl from 37% (v/v) concentrate and 10% formic acid (HCOOH) from 89% (v/v) concentrate (pH = 5) at 37°C. The success of complete decalcification was evaluated subjectively and experientially. The tissue was fixed in a circular tissue processor (Leica TP 1020, Germany) after decalcification, and then molded in paraffin blocks.

Serial tissue sections of 4 μm thickness (8 from each sample) were cut from paraffin molds in the mesiodistal direction. The sections were caught on a glass slide and placed at a temperature of 56–68°C (melting point of paraffin) for one hour, to fix the samples to the glass slide and dry them. The preparations were then stained with hematoxylin-eosin (HE) and Goldner trichrome staining. H&E was used for stereological measurements, and Goldner trichrome was used for bone mineralization detection.

Stereological measurements were performed to observe the difference in the representation of bone tissue and matrix cells in the CS and HA-CS groups. Microscopic preparations were analyzed by optical microscopy using an LM Leica microscope at magnifications ×10, ×40, ×100, ×200, and ×450. Pathohistological parameters were analyzed qualitatively, semiquantitatively, and quantitatively. Histomorphometric analysis was performed according to the cellularity and thickness of the newly formed tissue. Parameters were scored using a scoring system from 1 to 4, according to the modified criteria of Accorinte et al. [42].

2.1.1 Results

After the application of CS and HA-CS materials in the artificial furcation defects of the teeth of Vietnamese pigs, no inflammatory reaction was recorded in the periodontal and bone tissue of any sample (grade 1). No giant cells or microorganisms were found (score 1). A small number of material particles were detected in most of the CS and HA-CS group samples (grade 2).

The results of cytohistological and stereological analyzes of bone after implantation of CS and HA-CS materials in the furcation of porcine teeth are shown in **Tables 1** and **2**; and **Figures 1–6**.

The results showed that the volume and numerical density of osteocytes, as well as the number of osteocytes, was higher after implantation of HA-CS material than after implantation of CS material in the area of the tooth furcation, which represented a statistically significant difference. The volume density of the mineralized extracellular matrix in the bone tissue in the HA-CS group was higher compared to

Parameter (unit)	**CS**	**HA-CS**
Osteocyte volume density (mm^0)	0.129 ± 0.015	0.201 ± 0.018*
Osteocyte numerical density (mm^{-3})	1.333 ± 149	2.844 ± 199*
Number of osteocytes	7.046 ± 691	9.953 ± 809*
Volume density of the mineralized matrix (mm^0)	0.252 ± 0.078	0.339 ± 0.084
Bone marrow volume density (mm^0)	0.464 ± 0.052	0.296 ± 0.049
Bone marrow numerical density (mm^{-3})	2.125 ± 214	2.995 ± 237
Volume density of bone marrow mesenchymal cells (mm^0)	0.110 ± 0.019	0.177 ± 0.021
Numerical density of bone marrow mesenchymal cells (mm^{-3})	6.011 ± 715	7.908 ± 804*
Number of bone marrow mesenchymal cells	50.916 ± 1418	62.390 ± 1902
Volume density of bone marrow fibroblasts (mm^0)	0.127 ± 0.028	0.183 ± 0.035
Numerical density of fibroblasts of bone marrow cells (mm^{-3})	5.506 ± 422	7.116 ± 616*
Number of bone marrow fibroblasts	41.315 ± 1225	54.082 ± 1609
Volume density of blood capillaries (mm^0)	0.155 ± 0.033	0.164 ± 0.038
Numerical density of blood capillaries (mm^{-3})	1.042 ± 207	1.769 ± 219
Number of endothelial cells of blood capillaries	9.360 ± 647	10.912 ± 828

**Statistically significant difference for $p<0.05$.*

Table 1.
Values of stereological parameters of bone in the root perforation of Vietnamese pigs teeth with two types of materials CS and HA-CS (mean value±SD).

	Material	Thickness of the peridontium (μm)	Surface of the peridontium ($μm^2$)	Volume density of the peridontium (mm^0)
1.	CS	22.255 ± 2.818	11084.45 ± 1809.72	0.2315 ± 0.0085
2.	HA-CS	30.437 ± 2.995	9273.15 ± 1006.56	0.3204 ± 0.0092
t-test		p = 0.081295	p = 0.117409	p = 0.021673*
f-test		p = 0.194002	p = 0.318256	p = 0.041199*

**Statistically significant difference.*

Table 2.
Results of morphometric and stereological values of the periodontium in pig teeth with CS and HA-CS (mean value ± SD, p<0.05).

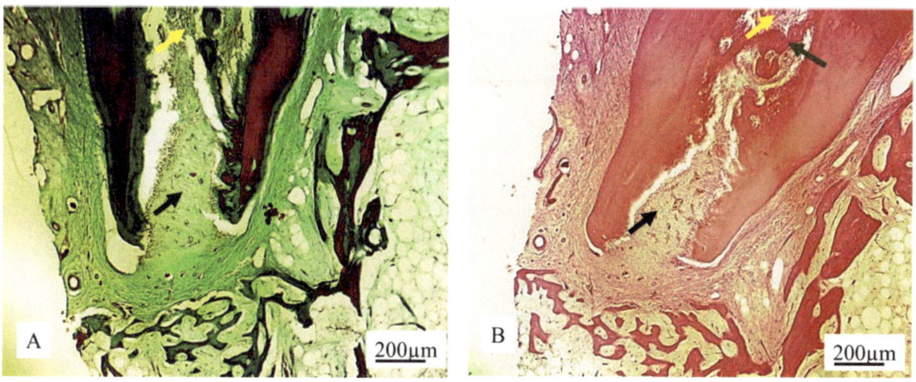

Figure 1.
Micrographs of histological sections of pig teeth: (A) CS, Goldner, and (B) HA-CS, H&E, applied material in the perforation area (yellow arrow), newly formed bone (black arrow), complete healing at the perforation site (green arrow), ×40.

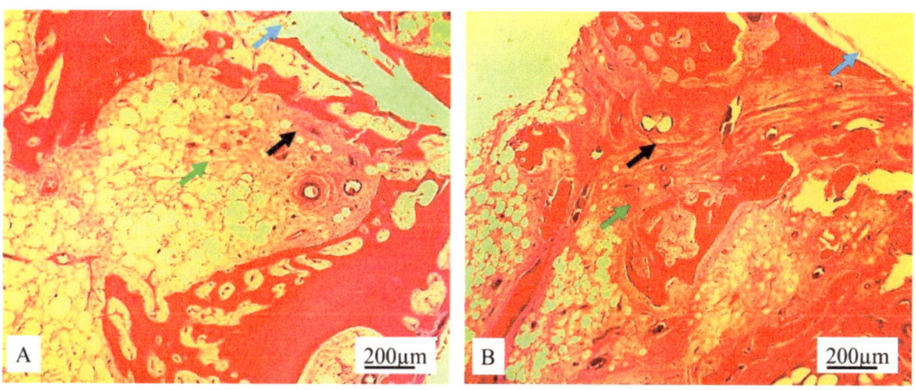

Figure 2.
Micrographs of histological sections of pig teeth: (A) CS and (B) HA-CS, histochemical technique Picrosirius red, applied material in the area of the furcation (blue arrow), newly formed bone (green arrow), collagen depots (black arrow), ×40.

the CS group. A higher percentage of newly formed bone was observed in the HA-CS group (25.66%) compared to the CS group. The mean bone marrow volume density was lower in the HA-CS group compared to the CS group, and the numerical bone

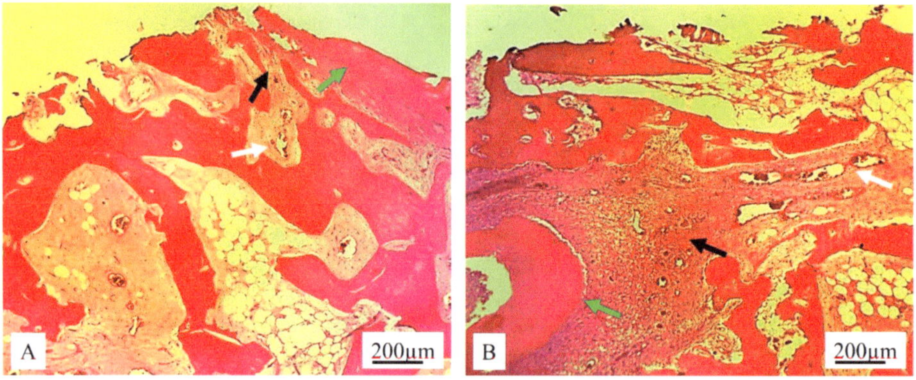

Figure 3.
Micrographs of histological sections of pig teeth: (A) CS and (B) HA-CS, histochemical technique Picrosirius red, periodontium (green arrow), newly formed bone (black arrow), blood vessels (white arrow), ×40.

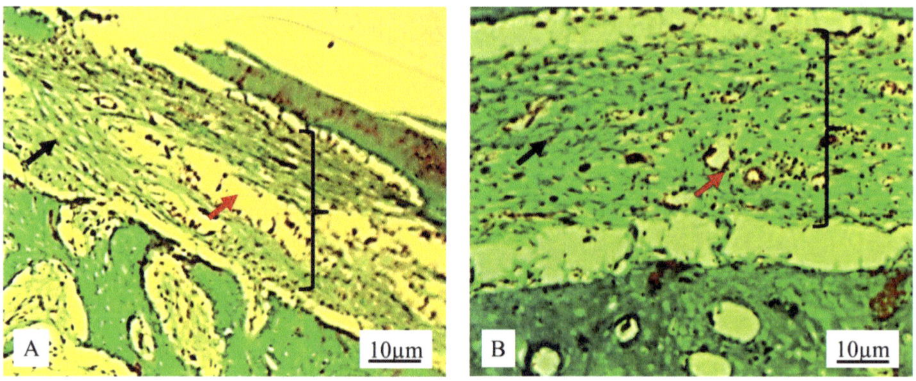

Figure 4.
Micrographs of histological sections of the peridontia of pig teeth: (A) CS, and (B) HA-CS, different width of periodontium (black bracket), blood vessels (red arrow), and peridontium (black arrow), Goldner, ×450.

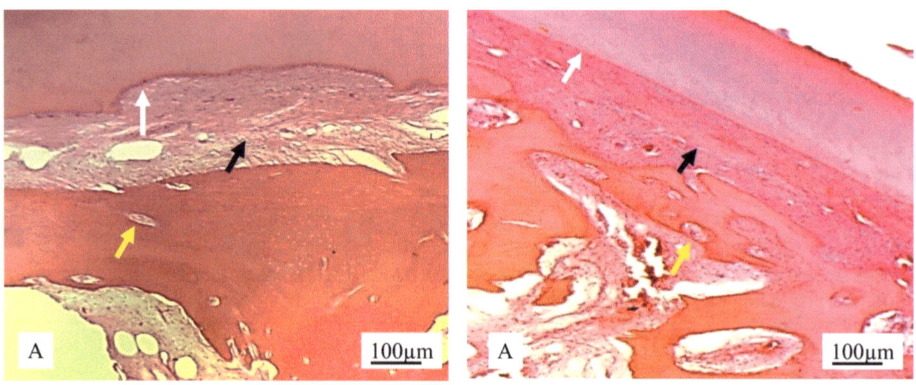

Figure 5.
Micrographs of histological sections of pig teeth: (A) CS, and (B) HA-CS, H&E, periodontium (white arrow), osteoblast activity surface (black arrow), and newly formed bone (yellow arrow), ×100.

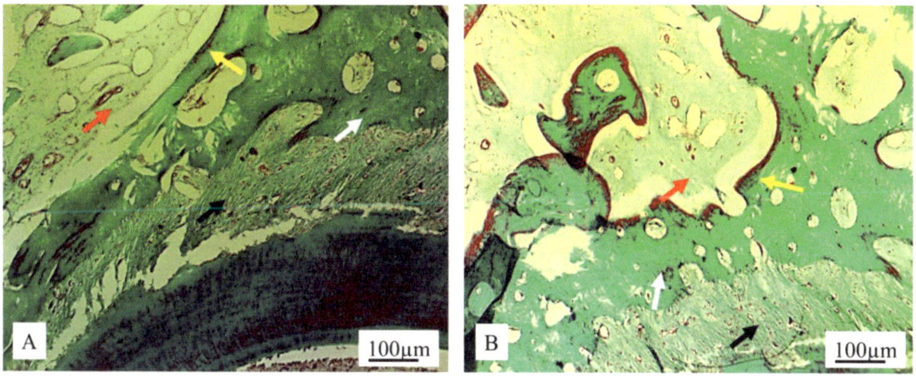

Figure 6.
Micrographs of histological sections of pig teeth: (A) CS, and (B) HA-CS, Goldner, remnants of applied materials (red arrow), periodontium (yellow arrow), newly formed bone (white arrow), and newly formed tendon tissue (black arrow), ×100.

marrow density was higher in the HA-CS group compared to the CS group. These data imply that the mitogenic effect led to an increase in the number of bone marrow cells and not to an increase in its volume in the bone tissue. This was the reason to make individual measurements of volume and numerical densities, as well as the number of mesenchymal cells and fibroblasts in the bone marrow.

The results of these measurements showed that the volume and numerical density, as well as the number of the mentioned cells in the bone marrow, were higher in the HA-CS group compared to the CS group. Also, less extracellular substance was observed in the same tissue in the bone marrow. Stereological parameters of blood capillaries showed a slight increase in values in the tissue of the HA-CS group compared to the CS group, which is a consequence of increased mitosis of all types of bone tissue cells.

Newly formed calcified tissue was observed in all samples after the application of both CS and HA-CS (**Figure 1**). In all samples of the HA-CS group, the implanted material was completely separated from the adjacent tissue by newly formed, properly structured, calcified continuous tissue (grade 1) (**Figure 1B**), whose thickness was 190–210 μm. Incomplete closure of the perforation by newly formed calcified tissue (green arrow) 125–160 μm thick is present in CS material in most samples. The newly formed calcified tissue in the CS group mostly had an irregular morphology (grade 2).

HA-CS performed significantly better than CS in terms of continuity and thickness of newly formed calcified tissue ($p = 0.008$).

Immunostaining for collagen (Picrosirius red) is a method by which, based on the detection of collagen, the quality of newly formed bone is determined. The results showed that the newly formed bone under the HA-CS material was of better quality and denser (**Figure 2**) and that there were more depots of extracellular collagen in the form of strips compared to the CS group (black arrow).

The newly formed bone was more regular and denser in contact with the periodontium in the HA-CS group than in the CS group (**Figures** 2 and **3**). A thin layer of periodontium (green arrow) is observed in most samples under the applied material (**Figure 3**). The activity of osteoblasts leading to new bone formation (black arrow) and the presence of newly formed blood vessels (white arrows) are also observed. Blood vessels are more numerous and larger in the HA-CS than in the CS group.

The results of morphometric and stereological measurements of the periodontium tissue are shown in **Table 2**; and **Figures 4–6**.

The thickness of the newly formed periodontium in the area of the furcation in the HA-CS group was 26.88% higher than in the CS group. The surface of the periodontium in the area of the furcation was 16.34% higher in the HA-CS group compared to the CS group. The volume density of the periodontium was 27.75% higher in HA-CS compared to CS, which was a statistically significant difference.

Histological and morphometric and stereological data show that the newly formed periodontal tissue was better and more regular in HA-CS material (**Figure 4**, black bracket) (**Table 2**). The connective tissue of the periodontium under the applied HA-CS material was more regular and dense (**Table 2**, **Figure 4**, black arrow), and the blood vessels were narrower and more numerous (red arrow). The volume density of the periodontium was statistically significantly higher ($p = 0.021673$) in the HA-CS group compared to the periodontium of the CS group. The blood vessels of the periodontium in the CS group were wider, dilated, with remnants of clustered erythrocytes.

Histological analysis shows that the newly formed periodontium in the HA-CS group is thicker compared to the CS group. Mesenchymal cells with osteoblastic differentiation were observed at the periphery of the newly calcified tissue. These cells are more numerous and fill the entire space between the periodontium and newly formed bone in the HA-CS material, while they are found in smaller numbers in the CS group (**Figure 5**).

The periodontium is histologically more regular, thicker, and more reactive to staining in the HA-CS group compared to CS. Newly formed bone (white arrow) is observed below the periodontium and the beginnings of tendon tissue formation (black arrow) are observed below it (**Figure 6**). Newly formed bone is histologically more regular and thicker, as well as tendon tissue which is thicker in teeth with HA-CS compared to CS.

2.2 Implantation of CS and HA-CS in root canals of rabbit teeth

Experimental research was carried out at the Institute of Surgery of the Faculty of Veterinary Medicine, University of Belgrade. Permission for experimental work with animals was obtained from the Ethics Committee of the Faculty of Dentistry, University of Belgrade, Serbia (Protocol No. 36/21/2013), conducted according to international standards ISO10993-2 (Requirements for animal welfare) and ISO 7405 [41].

Four rabbits from the genus Orictolagus cuniculus, aged 12 months and with an average weight of 4 kg, were included in the research.

Animals were kept in standard, individual cages, given ad libitum access to water, and standard rabbit chow. Daily monitoring of the animals was performed while the experiment lasted. Before the surgery, the animals were put under general anesthesia with Xylazine (2% Xylazine, Czech Republic) 35 mg/kg body weight and Ketamidor (100% Ketamidor 100 mg/ml, Richter Pharma AG, Austria) 5 mg/kg body weight.

The working field was disinfected with 5% tincture of iodine. Round diamond bur was used for preparing the class I cavities on the upper and lower central incisors. Access cavities were formed and coronary pulp tissue was removed with sterile, round, and carbide burs. Root canals were instrumented with K files #40 (VDV Gmbh, Germany) after extirpation of the radicular pulp and irrigated with 5 ml saline between each instrument. A new set of endodontic instruments was used for each animal. Then, the canals were dried with paper points and filled with freshly mixed material. Experimental and nanostructured cements, CS and HA-CS, were mixed with distilled water in a ratio of 2:1 [33]. The control material, mineral trioxide aggregate (White MTA, Angelus® Solu oes odontologicas, Londrina, Brazil) was mixed according to the manufacturer's instructions, in a powder-to-liquid ratio of 3:1. MTA was applied in the right maxillary incisors of all animals. In both mandibular incisors and left maxillary incisors of two animals were applied CS, HA-CS was applied in the left maxillary incisors and both mandibular incisors of remaining two animals. The materials were introduced with a lentulo spiral and condensed with a hand compactor into the root canals. The cavities were then closed with voice ionomer cement (GC FUJI VIII, GC Corporation, Tokyo, Japan). Postoperatively, the animals received subcutaneously an analgesic (Butorphanol, 10 mg/ml, Richter Pharma AG Austria), 0.1 mg/kg body weight, every 8 h for the next three days and an antibiotic (Baitril®, 25 mg/ml, KVP Pharma und Veterinar Produkte GmbH), 10 mg/kg body weight, daily for the next five days. After 28 days, animals were sacrificed by intravenous injection of 10 ml of pentobarbital solution (pentobarbital sodium salt 100 mg ml-1, Sigma-Aldrich Chemie GmbH, Steinheim, Germany).

The treated teeth together with the bone tissue of the upper or lower jaw were cut with a diamond disc in the form of block sections and fixed in 10% formalin after removing the soft tissues and separating the upper and lower jaw. The samples were decalcified in a decalcification solution: 8% HCl from 37% (v/v) concentrate and 10% formic acid (HCOOH) from 89% (v/v) concentrate (pH = 5) at 37°C. The success of complete decalcification was evaluated subjectively and experientially. The tissue was fixed in a circular tissue processor (Leica TP 1020, Germany) after decalcification and then molded in paraffin blocks.

Serial tissue sections (eight per sample) of 5 μm thickness were cut from paraffin blocks and stained with hematoxylin eosin (HE) according to standard procedure. Glass histological slides were analyzed with an optical microscope (Olympus 5 microscope) using the morphometric software package "Cell-B" (Olympus), at magnifications of 40x, 100x, and 200x, by an experienced pathologist who did not know the types of examined materials. Histological parameters were analyzed qualitatively (presence of inflammation, general tissue condition, continuity, and morphology of calcified tissue), semi-quantitatively (presence of giant cells, particles of material, and microorganisms), and quantitatively (intensity of inflammatory reaction, thickness of calcified tissue). Histomorphometric analysis was performed according to the cellularity and thickness of the calcified tissue. Parameters were scored using a scoring system from 1 to 4 according to the modified criteria of Accorinte et al. [42].

2.2.1 Results

Half of the samples showed no inflammatory reaction after CS material implantation (grade 1) (**Figure 7**). In two samples, inflammatory reactions were moderate (grade 3). In one sample, inflammatory reaction was pronounced (grade 4), with deep tissue infiltration of inflammatory cells and abscess formation (grade 3). Particles of implanted material were detected in all samples, but in different numbers (grades 2–4). Giant cells were detected in half of the samples—(grade 1), and giant cells were detected in the other half in small numbers (grade 2). Microorganisms were not detected in any sample.

The tissue was unchanged after implantation of the HA-CS material (grade 1) in most samples (**Figure 8**). Mild inflammatory reaction (grade 2) was detected in two samples (score 2). Material particles were detected in most samples (grade 2). Microorganisms and giant cells were not detected (grade 1).

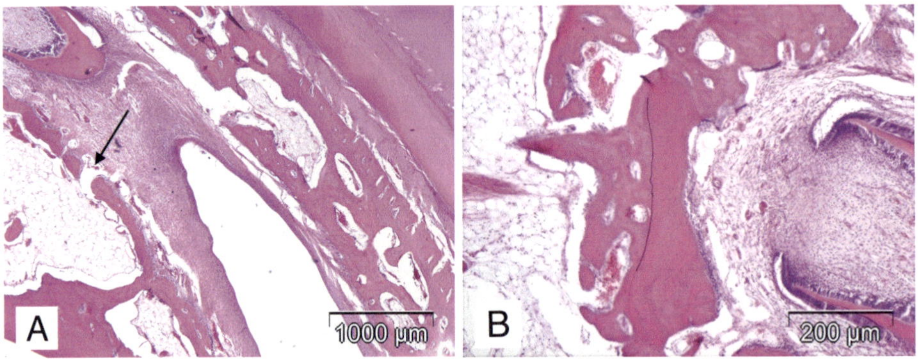

Figure 7.
CS. Photomicrograph of calcified tissue with proliferation of the connective tissue, moderate cellularity with slight macrophage infiltration. Discontinuous newly formed calcified tissue (black arrow) with a clear border between old and new osteoid (black line). Irregular structure of newly formed calcified tissue (HE, 200×).

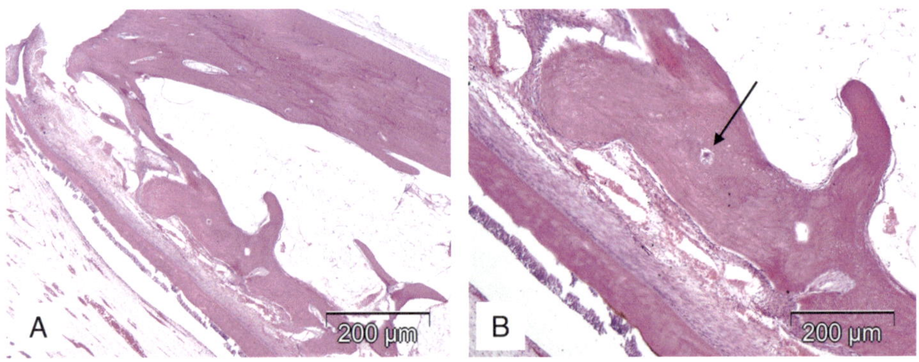

Figure 8.
HA-CS. Continuous calcified tissue with lamellar structure (HE, 40×). Calcified tissue with regular mineralization. Viable osteocyte is presented in newly formed bone (black arrows).

Different inflammatory reaction was observed after MTA implantation (grades 2–3), with inflammatory cells near the implanted material (grade 2) (**Figure 9**). Material particles were detected in all samples (grade 2). Few giant cells were found in most samples (grade 2). Microorganisms were not detected (grade 1).

There were no statistically significant differences in the intensity of inflammatory reactions between the tested materials. There were statistically significant differences between HA-CS and CS regarding the extent of inflammation ($p = 0.004$).

Newly formed calcified tissue was mostly irregular in morphology in samples with CS (score 2), deposited in a thickness greater than 250 µm (scores 1–2) in most samples, but discontinuous with foci of fibrovascular tissue (scores 2–3) (**Figures** 7A, B).

The implanted material was completely separated from the adjacent tissue by newly formed, regularly structured, and calcified continuous tissue in most samples with HA-CS (score 1). The thickness of the newly formed tissue varied between 150 and 250 µm (scores 1–2). Mesenchymal cells with osteoblastic differentiation were observed at the periphery of the newly calcified tissue (**Figures 8**A, B).

New calcified tissue was deposited in small amounts, up to 150 µm thick, in all samples with MTA (score 3). The newly formed calcified tissue was irregularly structured and discontinuous with foci of fibrovascular proliferation (scores 2–3) (**Figures 9**A, B).

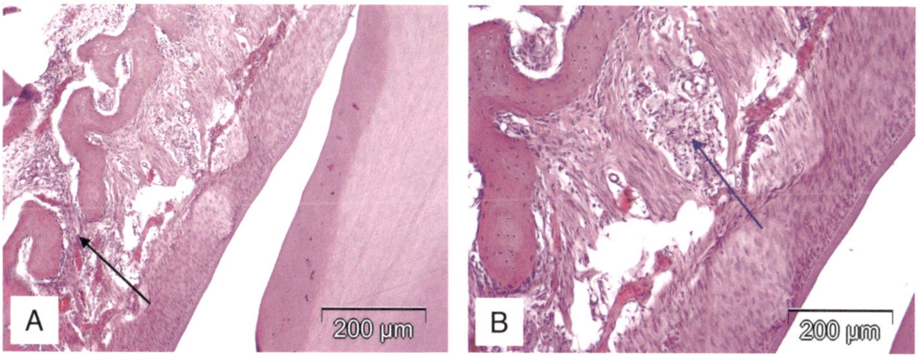

Figure 9.
MTA. Foci of fibrovascular proliferation (black arrow) in partially discontinuous newly formed calcified tissue (HE, 40×). Regular structure of calcified tissue with many osteocytes. Material particles (blue arrow) (HE, 200×).

HA-CS performed significantly better than MTA and CS in terms of continuity of newly formed calcified tissue ($p = 0.03$ and $p = 0.010$, respectively). There were significant differences in calcified tissue thickness between CS and MTA ($p = 0.004$) and between HA-CS and MTA ($p = 0.012$).

3. Discussion

The complex interaction between the material and the host tissue is best demonstrated by *in vivo* tests. These tests, in addition to biocompatibility, enable the evaluation of the biofunctionality of the material. In these two experimental studies, the effects of the materials were evaluated after their implantation in artificially created perforations in the furcation area of the teeth of Vietnamese pigs and application in the root canals of rabbit teeth.

In a rabbit study, the CS and HA-CS materials induced an inflammatory reaction of the periradicular tissue that was similar in intensity to the control material (MTA). Inflammatory reactions were rated as mild to moderate in most samples, indicating a good tolerance of the host tissue to the applied materials. These findings are consistent with the results of other authors who examined the biocompatibility of materials with similar chemical composition [42].

In another study on Vietnamese pigs, no inflammatory reaction was noted in any sample after implantation of CS and HA-CS in the furcation area of the tooth. The results of de Silva and the authors show that the inflammatory reaction is most intense in the first seven days after the application of the tested material and that the intensity of the inflammation decreases over time [43].

Inflammatory reactions after the application of calcium silicate cements are the result of the release of calcium hydroxide during the setting of the material. High pH causes local tissue necrosis with the development of local inflammatory reactions [44]. As a consequence of the alkaline pH, silicate cement induces the expression of proinflammatory cytokines (IL-6 and IL-8) [45]. It is known that tissue necrosis is the initiator of the mineralization process [46]. Some studies show that repair processes could start even without necrosis or acute inflammation [47]. As the material sets as a function of time, the amount of calcium hydroxide released from calcium silicate cements decreases [47]. By binding the material, favorable conditions are created for the beginning of the reparation process.

Although no statistically significant differences were found between CS, HA-CS, and MTA in the rabbit tissue regarding the inflammatory response, the tissue condition in the samples with HA-CS was rated as the best. This finding may be a consequence of the composition of such material. HA-CS consists mainly of hydroxyapatite with a slightly lower pH value than CS and MTA [35]. Lower pH values are thought to promote alkaline phosphatase activity but cause a smaller zone of surface necrosis compared to highly alkaline materials such as calcium silicate cements [48].

The low number of giant cells in samples with CS and MTA, or their absence in samples with HA-CS in both experiments, indicates a low activity of tissue histocytes and a good tissue tolerance to the implanted materials.

Newly formed calcified tissue was observed in all samples of the investigated materials in both experiments. It confirms that the examined nanostructured cements have an inductive potential. Previous studies also confirm the formation of mineralized tissue after the implantation of materials with the similar chemical composition [49].

CS and HA-CS belong to the group of bioactive materials that have the ability to release biologically active ions. The main soluble component of these cements is calcium hydroxide. It is released during the binding of the material. Considering that calcium silicate materials are characterized by a long bonding time, calcium hydroxide is released over several weeks [38]. Calcium hydroxide dissolves calcium and hydroxyl ions in contact with tissue and tissue fluids. The continuous release of calcium ions from the material is considered to be crucial for the induction of calcified tissue formation. In addition to its role in chemotaxis, calcium regulates cell proliferation, differentiation, and mineralization [39].

Calcium-releasing materials have been confirmed to induce the proliferation of periodontal fibroblasts, the growth and differentiation of pulp cells, osteoblasts, osteoblast-like cells, and cementoblasts [20].

The release of hydroxyl ions from implanted material is associated with tissue mineralization processes. An increase in alkaline phosphatase (ALP) occurs as a result of high pH, leading to the expression of growth factors and the formation of calcified tissue.

The tested materials also have Si ions in their composition, which influence the bioactivity of the material [50], and the proliferation and differentiation of cells similar to osteoblasts. High concentrations of Si ions (> 30 ppm) can inhibit osteoclast growth and resorption processes, but can also increase the level of ALP that participates in the mineralization of newly calcified tissue [51].

The result of the application of both nanostructured materials is a thicker layer of calcified tissue compared to MTA. Materials synthesized by the sol-gel method, such as CS and HA-CS in these studies, have improved bioactivity compared to the same materials obtained by other methods [52]. The topography of the surface of materials is related to their chemical composition and structure, and affects the activity of cells, especially their adhesion and vitality [47]. These results can be explained by the nanostructure of CS and HA-CS particles, which is similar to bone structure.

The newly formed calcified tissue, associated with HA-CS in both experiments, was continuous and without foci of vascularized fibroblast proliferation, which was not the case with MTA and CS. Unlike CS and MTA, HA-CS contains phosphate ions that could be related to this histological finding. Studies show that similar or better quality of calcified tissues are described after the application of calcium silicate cements containing phosphate ions, compared to pure calcium silicate cement [49]. The authors attributed these findings to the greater amount of phosphate ions available for hydroxyapatite formation. The present studies confirm that materials with hydroxyapatite have a greater potential for tissue mineralization than MTA [53].

There were no observed microorganisms in any sample of the implanted materials. The presence of microbes usually correlates with inadequate crown restorations and subsequent microleakage. GIC is material with good sealing properties and it may be the reason for the obtained result in this study. However, it must be emphasized that with this type of histochemical staining, microorganisms are difficult to detect and can be removed during tissue preparation for histological analysis.

4. Conclusion

The application of CS and HA-CS into the furcation defects of the teeth of Vietnamese pigs showed a complete absence of tissue inflammatory reaction, while this response was minimal after the application of these materials into the root canals of rabbit teeth, similar to the control MTA. CS and HA-CS were more effective than MTA in inducing the formation of calcified tissue after implantation in the root canals of rabbit teeth. The best organized newly formed calcified tissue was observed after the application of HA-CS in root canals of rabbits and root perforation of Vietnamese pigs. The present results serve as a solid basis for further biological studies of CS and HA-CS.

Conflict of interest

The authors have stated explicitly that there is no conflict of interest in connection with this chapter.

Author details

Marijana Popović Bajić[1]*, Violeta Petrović[1], Vanja Opačić Galić[1], Smiljana Paraš[2], Vukoman Jokanović[3] and Slavoljub Živković[1]

1 Department for Restorative Dentistry and Endodontics, School of Dental Medicine, University of Belgrade, Belgrade, Serbia

2 Faculty of Science and Mathematics, Department of Zoology, University of Banja Luka, Banja Luka, Republic of Srpska, Bosnia and Herzegovina

3 "Vinča" Institute of Nuclear Sciences, University of Belgrade, Belgrade, Serbia

*Address all correspondence to: dr.marijanapopovic@gmail.com

References

[1] Tsesis I, Fuss Z. Diagnosis and treatment of accidental root perforations. Endodontic Topics. 2006;**13**(1):95-107. DOI: 10.1111/j.1601-1546.2006.00213.x

[2] Estrela C, Biffi JC, Moura MS, Lopes HP. Treatment of endodontic failure. In: Estrela C, editor. Endodontic Science. 2nd ed. São Paulo: Artes Médicas; 2009. pp. 917-952

[3] Roda RS, Gettleman BH. Nonsurgical retreatment. In: Hargreaves KM, Berman LH, editors. Cohen's Pathways of the Pulp. 11th ed. St. Louis: Elservier; 2016. pp. 324-386

[4] Estrela C, Pécora JD, Estrela CRA, Guedes OA, Silva BS, Soares CJ, et al. Common operative procedural errors and clinical factors associated with root canal treatment. Brazilian Dental Journal. 2017;**28**(2):179-190. DOI: 10.1590/0103-6440201702451

[5] Ingle JI. A standardized endodontic technique utilizing newly designed instruments and filling materials. Oral Surgery, Oral Medicine, and Oral Pathology. 1961;**14**:83-91. DOI: 10.1016/0030-4220(61)90477-7

[6] Touré B, Faye B, Kane AW, Lo CM, Niang B, Boucher Y. Analysis of reasons for extraction of endodontically treated teeth: A prospective study. Journal of Endodontia. 2011;**37**(11):1512-1515. DOI: 10.1016/j.joen.2011.07.002

[7] Holland R, Otobani Filho JA, Souza V, Nery MJ, Bernabé PF, Dezan JE. Mineral trioxide aggregate repair of lateral root perforations. Journal of Endodontia. 2001;**27**(4):281-284.DOI:10.1097/00004770-200104000-00011

[8] Farzaneh M, Abitbol S, Friedman S. Treatment outcome in endodontics: The Toronto study. Phases I and II: Orthograde retreatment. Journal of Endodontia. 2004;**30**:627-633

[9] Eldeeb M, Tabibi A, Jensen JR. An evaluation of the use of amalgam, cavit and calcium hydroxide in the repair of furcation perforations. Journal of Endodontia. 1982;**8**:459-466

[10] Oswald R. Procedural accidents and their repair. Dental Clinics of North America. 1979;**23**:593-616

[11] Haghgoo R, Arfa S, Asgary S. Microleakage of CEM cement and ProRoot MTA as furcal perforation repair materials in primary teeth. Iranian Endodontic Journal. 2013;**8**:187-190

[12] Gutmann JL, Harrison JW. Posterior endodontic surgery: Anatomical considerations and clinical techniques. International Endodontic Journal. 1985;**18**:8-34

[13] Kakani AK, Veeramachaneni C, Majeti C, Tummala M, Khiyani L. A review on perforation repair materials. Journal of Clinical and Diagnostic Research. 2015;**9**(9):ZE09-ZE13. DOI: 10.7860/JCDR/2015/13854.6501

[14] Estrela C, Decurcio D, Rossi-Fedele G, Silva JA, Guedes OA, Borges AH, et al. Root perforations: A review of diagnosis, prognosis and materials. Brazilian Oral Research. 2018;**32**:133-146. DOI: 10.1590/1807-3107bor-2018.vol32.0073. Epub 18 Oct 2018

[15] Kakani AK, Veeramachaneni C. Sealing ability of three different root repair materials for furcation perforation repair: An *in vitro* study. Journal of Conservative Dentistry. 2020;**23**(1):62-65. DOI: 10.4103/JCD.JCD_371_19

[16] Silveira CM, Sánchez-Ayala A, Lagravère MO, Pilatti GL, Gomes OM. Repair of furcal perforation with mineral trioxide aggregate: Long-term follow-up of 2 cases. Journal of the Canadian Dental Association. 2008;**74**:729-733

[17] Felippe WT, Felippe MC, Rocha MJ. The effect of mineral trioxide aggregate on the apexification and periapical healing of teeth with incomplete root formation. International Endodontic Journal. 2006;**39**:2-9. DOI: 10.1111/j.1365-2591. 2005.01037.x

[18] Torabinejad M, Parirokh M, Dummer PMH. Mineral trioxide aggregate and other bioactive endodontic cements: An updated overview—Part I: Vital pulp therapy. International Endodontic Journal. 2018;**51**:177-205

[19] Torabinejad M, Parirokh M, Dummer PMH. Mineral trioxide aggregate and other bioactive endodontic cements: An updated overview—Part II: Other clinical applications and complications. International Endodontic Journal. 2018;**51**:284-317

[20] Silva LAB, Pieroni KAMG, Nelson-Filho P, et al. Furcation perforation. Periradicular tissue response to biodentine as a repair material by histopathologic and indirect immunofluorescence analyses. Journal of Endodontia. 2017;**43**:1137-1142

[21] Kum KY, Kim EC, Yoo YJ. Et al: Trace metal contents of three tricalcium silicate materials: MTA angelus, micro mega MTA and bioaggregate. International Endodontic Journal. 2014;**47**:704-710

[22] Camilleri J. Hydratation characteristics of calcium silicate cements with alternative radiopacifiers used as root-end filling materials. Journal of Endodontia. 2010;**36**:502-508

[23] Ramos JC, Palma PJ, Nascimento R, et al. 1-year in vitro evaluation of tooth discoloration induced by 2 calcium silicate-based cements. Journal of Endodontia. 2016;**42**:1403-1407

[24] Camilleri J, Sorrentino F, Damidot D. Investigation of the hydration and bioactivity of radiopacified tricalcium silicate cement, Biodentine and MTA angelus. Dental Materials. 2013;**29**:580-593

[25] Parirokh M, Torabinejad M. Mineral trioxide aggregate: A comprehensive literature review—Part III: Clinical applications, drawbacks and mechanism of action. Journal of Endodontia. 2010;**36**:400-413

[26] Zhao Q, Qian J, Zhou H, Yuan Y, Mao Y, Liu C. In vitro osteoblast-like and endothelial cells response to calcium silicate/calcium phosphate cement. Biomedical Materials. 2010;**5**:1-8

[27] Jokanović V. Nanomedicina najveći izazov 21. Vekas: Data Status; 2012. p. 180

[28] Gui C, Dai X, Cui D. Advances of nanotechnology applied to biosensors. Nano Biomedicine & Engineering. 2011;**3**(4):260-273

[29] Fan JP, Kalia P, Di Silvio L, Huang J. In vitro response of human osteoblasts to multi-step sol-gel derived bioactive glass nanoparticles for bone tissue engineering. Materials Science and Engineering: C. 2014;**36**:206-214

[30] Chenab F, Zhub Y, Wub J, et al. Nanostructured calcium phosphates: Preparation and their application in biomedicine. Nano Biomedicine & Engineering. 2012;**4**(1):41-49

[31] Saghiri MA, Godoy FG, Gutmann JL, Lotfi M, Asatourian A, Sheibani N, et al. The effect of pH on solubility of nano-modified endodontic cements. Journal of Conservative Dentistry. 2014;**17**:13-17

[32] De Deus G, Canabarro A, Alves G, Linhares A, Senne MI, Granjeiro JM. Optimal cytocompatibility of a bioceramic nanoparticulate cement in primary human mesenchymal cells. Journal of Endodontia. 2009;**35**:1387-1390

[33] Jokanović V, Čolović B, Jokanović B, Živković S. Superplastic, quick-bonding endodontic mixtures and their hydration. International Journal of Applied Ceramic Technology. 2015;**12**(S2):E83-E91

[34] Opačić-Galić V, Petrović V, Živković S, et al. New nanostructural biomaterials based on active calcium silicate systems and hydroxyapatite:Characterization and genotoxicity in human peripheral blood lymphocytes. International Endodontic Journal. 2013;**46**:506-516

[35] Petrović V, Opačić Galić V, Jokanović V, Jovanović M, Basta Jovanović G, Živković S. Biocompatibility of a new nanomaterial based on calcium silicate implanted in subcutaneous connective tissue of rats. Acta Veterinaria-Beograd. 2012;**62**:697-708

[36] Opačić-Galić V, Petrović V, Jokanović V, Živković S. Histological evaluation of tissue reactions to newly synthetized calcium silicate-and-hydroxyapatite-based bioactive materials-In vivo study. Srpski Arhiv za Celokupno Lekarstvo. 2017;**145**:370-377

[37] Petrović V, Opačić-Galić V, Živković S, Nikolić B, Danilović V, Miletić V, et al. Biocompatibility of new nanostructural materials based on active silicate systems and hydroxyapatite: in vitro and in vivo study. International Endodontic Journal. 2015;**48**(10):966-975. DOI: 10.1111/iej.12391. [Epub 2014 Nov 5]

[38] Sarkar NK, Caicedo R, Ritwik P, Moiseyeva R, Kawashima I. Physicochemical basis of the biologic properties of mineral trioxide aggregate. Journal of Endodontia. 2005;**31**:97-100

[39] Gandolfi MG, Ciapetti G, Perut F, et al. Biomimetic calcium-silicate cements aged in simulated body solutions. Osteoblast response and analyses of apatite coating. Journal of Applied Biomaterials & Biomechanics. 2009;**7**:160-170

[40] Jokanović V, Cicović B, Prokić BB, Tomanović N, Popović Bajić M, Živković S. Subchronic systemic toxicity of new endodontic material based on calcium hydroxyapatite and calcium silicates. Advances Mater Science and Engineering. 2018;**2018**:6. Article ID: 8493439. DOI: 10.1155/2018/8493439

[41] Opačić Galić V, Petrović V, Popović Bajić M, Jokanovič V, Živkovič S, Nikolić B, et al. Physical properties and biocompatibility of Nanostructural biomaterials based on active calcium silicate systems and hydroxyapatite. In: Chaughule RS, editor. Dental Applications of Nanotechnology. Vol. Chapter 13. Switzerland AG: Springer Nature; 2018. pp. 247-271. DOI: 10.1007/978-3-319-97634-1_13

[42] Accorinte Mde L, Holland R, Reis A, Bortoluzzi MC, Murata SS, Dezan E, et al. Evaluation of mineral trioxide aggregate and calcium hydroxide cement as pulp-capping agents in human teeth. Journal of Endodontia. 2008;**34**:1-6

[43] da Silva GF, Guerreiro-Tanomaru JM, Sasso-Cerri E, Tanomaru-Filho M, Cerri PS. Histological and histomorphometrical evaluation of furcation perforations filled with MTA, CPM and ZOE. International Endodontic Journal. 2011;**44**(2):100-110. DOI: 10.1111/j.1365-2591.2010.01803.x. Epub 2010 Oct 12

[44] Tran XV, Gorin C, Willig C, et al. Effect of a calcium-silicate-based restorative cement on pulp repair. Journal of Dental Research. 2012;**91**:1166-1171

[45] Chen CC, Shie MY, Ding SJ. Human dental pulp cell response to new calcium silicate-based endodontic materials. International Endodontic Journal. 2011;**44**:836-842

[46] Sangwan P, Sangwan A, Duha J, Rohilla A. Tertiary dentinogenesis with calcium hydroxide: A review of proposed mechanisms. International Endodontic Journal. 2013;**46**:3-19

[47] Anselme K. Osteoblast adhesion on biomaterials. Biomaterials. 2000;**21**:667-681

[48] Silva EJNL, Rosa TP, Herrera DR, Jacinto RC, Gomes BPFA, Zaia AA. Evaluation of cytotoxicity and physicochemical properties of calcium silicate-based endodontic sealer MTA Fillapex. Journal of Endodontia. 2013;**39**:274-277

[49] Zarrabi MH, Javidi M, Jafarian AH, Joushan B. Histologic assessment of human pulp response to capping with mineral trioxide aggregate and a novel endodontic cement. Journal of Endodontia. 2010;**36**:1778-1781

[50] Huan Z, Chang J. Calcium-phosphate-silicate composite bone cement: Self-setting properties and in vitro bioactivity. Journal of Materials Science: Materials in Medicine. 2009;**20**:833-841

[51] Pietak AM, Reid JW, Stott MJ, Sayer M. Silicon substitution in the calcium phosphate bioceramics. Biomaterials. 2007;**28**:4023-4032

[52] Li P, de Groot K. Better bioactive ceramics through sol-gel process. Journal of Sol-Gel Science and Technology. 1994;**2**:797-801

[53] Zhang S, Yang X, Fan M. Bioaggregate and iRoot BP plus optimize the proliferation and mineralization ability of human dental pulp cells. International Endodontic Journal. 2013;**46**:923-929

Chapter 6

The Relationship of Some Neurodegenerative Diseases with Endoplasmic Reticulum Stress and Histopathological Changes in These Diseases: An Overview

Adem Kara, Volkan Gelen and Hülya Kara

Abstract

The endoplasmic reticulum (ER) is an organelle responsible for protein production in the cell and provides hemostasis in the cell. ER stress is stimulated by folded proteins, while the unfolded protein response (UPR) creates a response to ER stress and provides the cell survival. UPR modulation in mammals is provided with three major ER stress sensors, including transmembrane kinase 1, protein kinase-like ER kinase, and activating transcription factor 6. Because neurons are susceptible to misfolded proteins, severe or prolonged ER stress activates apoptotic cell death signals in the cell. Neurodegenerative diseases characterized by this condition are Alzheimer's disease, Parkinson's disease, amyotrophic lateral sclerosis, and Huntington's disease, characterized by the accumulation and aggregation of misfolded proteins. In addition, ER stress can lead to depression, schizophrenia, sleep disruption, and post-traumatic stress disorders. Neurons are highly susceptible to protein misfolding and apoptotic cell death. For this reason, UPR modulation contributes to preventing the neurodegenerative process in cells with misfolded protein folding. The relationship between ER stress, UPR, and neuropathology is significant for understanding this process. This section will discuss the effects of ER stress between UPR modulation and neurodegenerative disorders, and the histopathological changes in the mentioned neurodegenerative diseases will be mentioned.

Keywords: ER stress, neurodegenerative disease, apoptosis, histopathology, neuropathology

1. Introduction

The endoplasmic reticulum (ER) is an organelle consisting of various structures in the form of interconnected channels and sacs in the cell [1]. The ER has various functions in the cell, such as being responsible for lipid synthesis, carbohydrate metabolism, calcium storage, and protein trafficking. Since it performs these tasks, it is of great importance that the ER function is normal [2]. Excess nutrient intake or exceeding the working capacity of the ER for various reasons causes the accumulation of misfolded proteins in the ER, and thus the deterioration of ER homeostasis due to difficulties in meeting the demand [3]. As a result of this situation, a situation called ER stress occurs. Recently, the number of studies on this subject has been increasing due to the prevalence of ER stress. If ER stress is excessive, apoptosis occurs because the cell cannot adapt [4]. It has been determined that ER stress triggers many diseases in the organism. These diseases include obesity, diabetes, ischemia-reperfusion diseases, and neurodegenerative diseases [5]. Neurodegenerative diseases are very diverse and affect human health negatively [6]. In addition, the first is an attractive topic because the treatment of neurodegenerative diseases is limited [7]. Parkinson's, Alzheimer's, and Huntington's are among these harvests [8, 9]. In the diseases mentioned, some histopathological changes occur in various parts of the brain. Our aim in this study is to describe the definition of ER stress, the mechanisms of ER stress, the relationship of ER stress with neurodegenerative diseases, and the specific histopathological changes that occur in these diseases.

2. Endoplasmic reticulum stress

As we mentioned earlier, increased metabolic demand, infection, hypoxia, excessive lipid accumulation, genetic disorders, and various toxins can disrupt ER homeostasis and cause ER stress due to misfolded or unfolded protein accumulation [6]. To reduce ER stress, a signaling pathway called the unfolded protein response (UPR) is activated, which slows protein synthesis and increases protein degradation [7, 8]. Activated UPR creates a stress response via protein kinase R (PKR)-like endoplasmic reticulum kinase (PERK) [9, 10], inositol-requiring enzyme 1 (IRE-1) [10–12], and activating transcription factor 6 (ATF-6) [13, 14]. IRE1 acts by activating Jun N-terminal kinase (JNK) [15]. ATF-6 increases the expression of the X-box binding protein 1 (XBP-1s) factor in the nucleus [16]. XBP-1s binds to some genes containing DNA regions, and in ER expansion, folding capacity is increased. It stimulates the transcription of genes involved in the ER-related degradation pathway and the activation of the ER-related degradation pathway, and the demand load on the ER is alleviated. With this mechanism, unfolded proteins are degraded. When this function fails, the ER activates the nuclear factor kappa B (NF-kB) to produce a signal in the cell [15]. After this signal, some apoptotic genes are stimulated and apoptosis is triggered by the stimulated genes.

2.1 Activation of PERK (protein kinase R (PKR)-like endoplasmic reticulum kinase)

PERK activation plays an important role in ER stress [17]. PERK has a specific binding site for GRP78, a chaperone involved in protein folding known as 78-kDa glucose-regulated protein (GRP78/BIP) [18]. After unfolded or misfolded proteins accumulate in the lumen, GRP78 separates from PERK and causes PERK to oligomerize [19]. Then, PERK activates itself. Then, PERK phosphorylates eukaryotic initiation factor 2 (eIF2α) [20]. While eIF2α is phosphorylated, it remains bound to eIF2B, which acts as GEF, thus preventing the formation of the translation initiation complex eIF2α/GTP/Met-tRNAi [21]. Phosphorylation of eIF2α under ER stress stimulates the translation of the transcription factor ATF-4, which plays a role in the ER stress response [18].

2.2 Activation of ATF-6 (activating transcription factor-6)

ATF-6 is a trans-membrane protein involved in ER stress [22]. After protein folding in the ER is inhibited, ATF-6 migrates to the Golgi apparatus. GRP78 is involved in this event [23]. There are GLS1 and GLS2 structures on ATF-6, which are involved in adhesion to the Golgi [24]. When GRP78 is bound to GLS1, it retains ATF-6 in the ER membrane [25]. If there is unfolded protein in the lumen, GRP78 dissociates from GLS1, and thus GLS2 is activated and migrates to ATF-6 Golgi [13]. In the Golgi, the transmembrane region of ATF-6 is cut, and eventually, the systolic bZIP region of ATF-6 travels to the nucleus and stimulates the transcription of XBP-1 [14]. The XBP-1s form of XBP-1 stimulates the transcriptional responses of the UPR. Thus, it reduces long-term ER stress [25].

2.3 Activation of IRE-1 (inositol-requiring enzyme 1)

IRE-1 is an ER transmembrane protein. In the ER stress state, IRE-1 is activated due to the cleavage of GRP78 and stimulates XBP-1 activation [26]. This stimulates the activation of XBP-1 s. XBP-1 s play a role in the differentiation of cells by increasing the transcription of genes responsible for ER expansion so that cells can respond to the increased demands of protein synthesis and modification [15]. XBP-1s travels to the nucleus and upregulates the transcription of genes involved in phospholipid synthesis, which drives ER-related degradation and expansion [27]. It also plays a role in the activation of IRE-1 and the activation of the JNK signaling pathway [28]. IRE-1 interacts with TNF receptor-associated factor 2 (TRAF2), activating its downstream signaling. TRAF2 then binds to ASK1, and ASK1 phosphorylates and activates JNK [26]. This effect of IRE-1 provides a bridge between ER stress, growth factors, and mitogens [15] (**Figure 1**).

2.4 ER functions and relations with organelles

The endoplasmic reticulum (ER) is a cytoplasmic organelle responsible for cytoplasmic protein synthesis [30]. The ER has many vital cellular functions, such as lipid and steroid synthesis, Ca2+ homeostasis and storage, carbohydrate metabolism, and protein synthesis [31]. With these features, the ER provides internal connection and coordination with other organelles and many proteins and physical structures in the cell. Therefore, they are in multiple contacts with all membrane-bound organelles, including the ER, plasma membrane (PM), mitochondria, Golgi, endosomes, and peroxisomes [30].

2.5 ER and plasma membrane (PM)

The ER acts as a Ca2+ store in the cell and has dynamic communication with the PM. Contact sites between ER and PM play a role in Ca2+ exchange. At ER-PM junctions, stromal interacting molecule (STIM) proteins sense a decrease in ER Ca2+ levels, undergo a conformational change along the ER that repositions tubular structures to ER-PM, and directly activate Orai, the pore-forming component of Ca2 + −. The release-activated Ca2 + (CRAC) channel triggers channel opening and Ca2+ influx [32]. In addition, ER-PM contact sites are important for phosphatidylinositol metabolism, particularly for the regulation of the lipid signaling molecule phosphatidylinositol 4-phosphate (PI4P) [30].

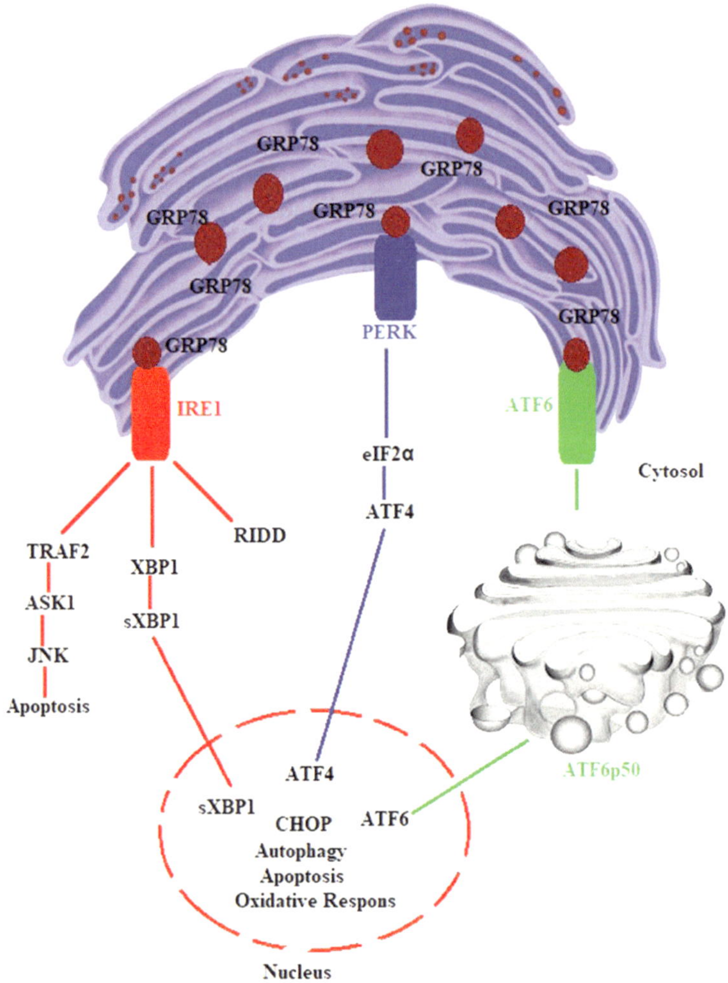

Figure 1.
Effective pathways in the ER stress response [29].

2.6 ER and mitochondria

Considering the relationship between the endoplasmic reticulum and mitochondria, there is a membrane that provides the connection between the ER and the mitochondria [30]. This membrane has been named the mitochondria-associated ER membrane (MAM). Communication between the ER and the mitochondria is provided by this membrane. This communication is very important for the survival of the cell. Many functions such as lipid transfer, autophagosome formation, mitochondrial fission, Ca2+ homeostasis, and apoptosis are regulated by this communication [33]. In this contact zone, calcium influx occurs into the intermembrane space and the mitochondrial matrix. It has been stated that changes in Ca2+ levels occur in case of disturbance in the regulation of this flow, thus affecting apoptosis, mitochondrial division, and motility, and altering the activity of mitochondrial Ca2+ binding proteins [34]. As a result, ER and mitochondrial communication disorders lead to a number of problems such as mitochondrial damage, Ca2+ dyshomeostasis, ER stress, defects in lipid metabolism, autophagy, decreased respiratory chain activity, and oxidative phosphorylation [35]. It has been determined that the communication disorder between these two organelles plays an important role in the regulation of neurological activity. It has been determined that the relationship between these organs is impaired in Alzheimer's, Parkinson's, and Huntington's disease [36].

3. ER stress and the unfolded protein response (UPR)

The ER is the main region in the cell where protein synthesis and post-synthesis changes take place, where newly synthesized proteins are folded and combined. The ER is extremely sensitive to many factors that will affect this function [37]. In case of any problem, misfolded or unfolded proteins begin to accumulate in the cytoplasm. When the protein concentration accumulated in the cytoplasm increases, the ER cannot cope with this load, and this causes the functioning to be worse [38]. Eukaryotic cells can adapt by reducing the rate of protein synthesis, upregulating the expression of genes encoding chaperones and other proteins that prevent polypeptide aggregation, and disrupting accumulated misfolded proteins. This set of cellular responses is obtained after activation of an integrated intracellular signaling cascade: the "Unfolded Protein Response" (UPR) [39]. The UPR is regulated by three sensor proteins known as PERK (PKR-like ER kinase), IRE1_ (inositol-requiring transmembrane kinase/endoribonuclease 1), and ATF6 (activating transcription factor 6). These proteins are associated with BiP or GRP78 (78 KDa glucose-regulated protein) and therefore remain inactive [29]. BiP is released under ER stress, and the response is shaped by further dimerization and autophosphorylation of PERK and IRE1 [40, 41]. The UPR cascade is activated after regulated intramembrane proteolysis of another regulatory sensor protein, ATF6, against the UPR [42] (**Figure 2**).

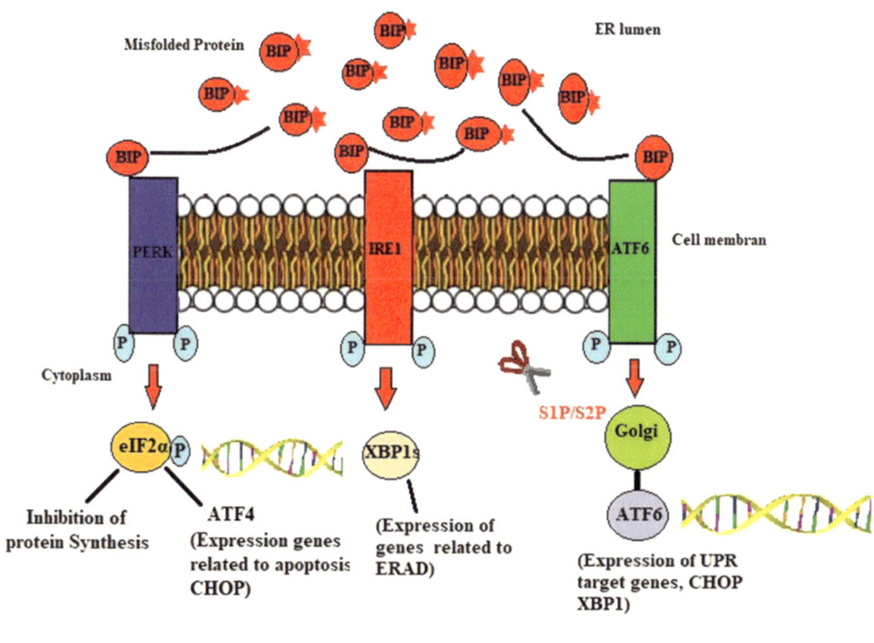

Figure 2.
The UPR. UPR is controlled by three sensor proteins [43].

4. Endoplasmic reticulum (ER) stress response and histopathological changes in Parkinson's disease

Parkinson's disease is a neuropathological disease involving the degeneration of dopaminergic neurons in the substantia nigra followed by loss of their terminals in the striatum [44]. The main clinical manifestations are resting tremor, bradykinesia, rigidity, and postural reflex dysfunction [44]. Currently, the cause of nigral degeneration, which is responsible for the development of the symptoms of this disease, is unknown. However, considering the studies, it is thought that hereditary predisposition, environmental toxins, and aging play an important role in this process and multifactorial causes come to the fore in etiopathogenesis. Various studies have shown that ER stress plays an essential role in the pathophysiology of Parkinson's [45]. ER stress occurs when protein aggregates and fibril accumulation in the Parkin cell with increased ROS in Parkinson's disease. In a study, it was reported that ER stress occurred in the cell culture medium. In another study, UPR components such as transcriptional factors and CHOP and ER chaperones in neurons cause damage to cells [45, 46]. It has also been stated that IRE, PERK, and ER stress kinase phosphorylation, which are involved in ER stress, play a role in Parkinson's and cause the degeneration of dopaminergic neurons [47]. Again, as a result of some studies, it has been reported that 6-OHDA and MPP+ applied to create experimental Parkinson's show their effects by triggering the UPR increase in neurons.

Characteristic features of Parkinson's disease include loss of neurons in certain areas of the brain region called the substantia nigra and extensive accumulation of intracellular protein (alpha-synuclein) [48]. While the loss of pigmented dopaminergic neurons in the substantia nigra and accumulation of α-synuclein in neurons are not specific for Parkinson's disease, these two major neuropathologies, when observed together, are specific for definitive diagnosis of idiopathic Parkinson's disease [49, 50].

5. Endoplasmic reticulum (ER) stress response and histopathological changes in Alzheimer's disease

Alzheimer's disease is the most common type of dementia. It is a progressive disease that begins with mild memory loss, possibly leading to loss of the ability to maintain speech and react to the environment [51]. Alzheimer's disease involves parts of the brain that control thought, memory, and language. As a result of studies on Alzheimer's, he stated that ER stress plays a vital role in the pathogenesis of Alzheimer's [52, 53]. Some studies determined that Ca homeostasis and accumulation of phosphorylated tau protein and intracellular amyloid-β play an important role in this disease. Again, some studies have shown that pPERK, pIRE1, and elF2α, which are the kinases of the UPR, are increased in the hippocampus and brain tissue neurons of Alzheimer's patients [54]. Again, PERK, eIF2α, and p38 MAPK activation associated with the presence of tau protein were observed in Alzheimer's patients. These findings clearly demonstrated the relationship between tau proteins in neurons and ER stress. In some studies, it has been stated that Alzheimer's disease increases as a result of cerebral ischemia or stroke. This is a clear indication that aging impairs the folded protein response by disrupting ER homeostasis due to oxidative stress and plays a role in the pathogenesis of the disease. Some studies on the UPR have reported increased levels of BIP/GRP78, protein kinase, and PERK in the brain of Alzheimer's patients [55].

The ER stress-mediated inflammatory response has an important role in Alzheimer's disease pathogenesis. The inflammatory response is normally triggered by the activation of inflammatory receptors, including TLRs (toll-like receptors) and NLRs (NOD-like receptors). These pattern recognition receptors transduce the signaling mostly via the NF-κB pathway and trigger the inflammatory response [56]. Additionally, the ER stress-mediated inflammatory response has a role in the pathogenesis of some diseases [57]. In obesity, ER stress can induce an inflammatory response and cause peripheral insulin resistance [58], and in the liver, ER stress can trigger the systemic inflammatory response and cause damage [59]. In neurodegenerative diseases, inflammatory processes are initiated by the maturation of the IL-1 cytokines called as inflammasomes [60].

Histopathologically senile amyloid in Alzheimer's disease plaques (SAP), neurofibrillary flock (NF) formation, loss of synapsneurons, and marked atrophy in the brain are detected [51]. The formation of senile plaques is the most important histopathological finding of the disease. It is a symptom of the disease and is seen especially in the amygdala, hippocampus, and neocortex. On the other hand, NF is required for the definitive diagnosis of AD [52]. And the detection of SPs is necessary but not sufficient. Both lesions occur both in normal aging and in some and can be seen in other neurodegenerative diseases. AD for the definitive diagnosis of NFY and SAP is a certain neuroanatomical. They must be shown to be in the distribution and in certain quantities [53].

6. Endoplasmic reticulum (ER) stress response and histopathological changes in Huntington's disease

Huntington's disease is a progressive and fatal neurodegenerative disease, and the mechanism that causes neuronal apoptosis has not been fully elucidated [61]. Studies have shown that ER stress, which occurs as a result of misfolded protein accumulation, which may contribute to neuronal loss, may play a role [62]. Although different studies have shown a role for the UPR in HD, the evidence is inconclusive [63]. In a study, RAB5A, HMGB1, CTNNB1, DNM1, TUBB, TSG101, EEF2, DYNC1H1, SLC12A5, ATG5, AKT1, CASP7, and SYVN1 genes were identified, which would suggest a potential link between UPR and Huntington's disease [64, 65]. A significant association was found in the length of the polyglutamine pathway of Huntington, which is a critical determinant of disease onset in human HD patients and points to the UPR as a promising target for therapeutic intervention [66].

The most affected region in terms of histopathological changes in HD is the striatal region. However, it was determined that gray and white matter were affected in cortical and noncortical areas. In addition, aggregates/inclusions are characteristic histopathological markers of HD.

7. Conclusion

As a result, the accumulation of unfolded or misfolded proteins in the cytosol under ER stress is an important mechanism in the occurrence of cell damage. PERK IRE1, and ATF6, which sense this protein folding response, play an important role in shaping the cellular pathway. In addition, the relationship between ER stress and mitochondria is important in the maintenance of cellular response. ER stress plays an important role in the pathogenesis of many neurodegenerative diseases such as Parkinson's, Alzheimer's, and Huntington's. Knowing the histopathological changes seen in these diseases is very important in the diagnosis of the disease. The role of misfolded or unfolded protein response in ER stress in neurodegenerative diseases, and the histopathological changes in these diseases will help to develop therapeutics for neurodegenerative diseases.

Author details

Adem Kara[1*], Volkan Gelen[2] and Hülya Kara[3]

1 Faculty of Science, Department of Molecular Biology and Genetics, Erzurum Technical University, Erzurum, Turkiye

2 Faculty of Veterinary Medicine, Department of Physiology, Kafkas University, Kars, Turkiye

3 Faculty of Veterinary Medicine, Department of Anatomy, Atatürk University, Erzurum, Turkiye

*Address all correspondence to: ademkara36@gmail.com

References

[1] Wu J, Kaufman RJ. From acute ER stress to physiological roles of the unfolded protein response. Cell Death and Differentiation. 2006;**13**:374-384

[2] Ron D, Walter P. Signal integration in the endoplasmic reticulum unfolded protein response. Nature Reviews. Molecular Cell Biology. 2007;**8**:519-529

[3] Lee AS. The glucose-regulated proteins: Stress induction and clinical applications. Trends in Biochemical Sciences. 2001;**26**:504-510

[4] Ledoux S, Yang R, Friedlander G, et al. Glucose depletion enhances P-glycoprotein expression in hepatoma cells: Role of endoplasmic reticulum stress response. Cancer Research. 2003;**63**:7284-7290

[5] Xu C, Bailly-Maitre B, Reed JC. Endoplasmic reticulum stress: Cell life and death decisions. The Journal of Clinical Investigation. 2005;**115**:2656-2664

[6] Caughey B, Lansbury PT. Protofibrils, pores, fibrils, and neurodegeneration: Separating the responsible protein aggregates from the innocent bystanders. Annual Review of Neuroscience. 2003;**26**:267-298

[7] Cavedo E, Lista S, Khachaturian Z, et al. The road ahead to cure Alzheimer's disease: Development of biological markers and neuroimaging methods for prevention trials across all stages and target populations. The Journal of Prevention of Alzheimer's Disease. 2014;**1**(3):181-202

[8] Cho KJ, Lee BI, Cheon SY, et al. Inhibition of apoptosis signal-regulating kinase 1 reduces endoplasmic reticulum stress and nuclear huntingtin fragments in a mouse model of Huntington disease. Neuroscience. 2009;**163**(4):1128-1134

[9] Chung CY, Khurana V, Auluck PK, et al. Identification and rescue of α-synuclein toxicity in Parkinson patient–derived neurons. Science. 2013;**342**(6161):983-987

[10] Urano F, Bertolotti A, Ron D. Ire1 and efferent signaling from the endoplasmic reticulum. Journal of Cell Science. 2000;**113**:3697-3702

[11] Boot-Handford R, Briggs MD. The unfolded protein response and its relevance to connective tissue diseases. Cell and Tissue Research. 2010;**339**:197-211

[12] Acosta-Alvear D, Zhou Y, Blais A, et al. Xbp1 controls diverse cell type- and condition-specific transcriptional regulatory networks. Molecular Cell. 2007;**27**:53-66

[13] Haze K, Yoshida H, Yanagi H, et al. Mammalian transcription factor ATF6 is synthesized as a transmembrane protein and activated by proteolysis in response to endoplasmic reticulum stress. Molecular Biology of the Cell. 1999;**10**:3787-3799

[14] Haze K, Okada T, Yoshida H, et al. Identification of the G13 (cAMP-response-element-binding protein-related protein) gene product related to activating transcription factor 6 as a transcriptional activator of the mammalian unfolded protein response. The Biochemical Journal. 2001;**355**:19-28

[15] Gardner BM, Walter P. Unfolded proteins are Ire1- activating ligands that

directly induce the unfolded protein response. Science. 2011;**333**:1891-1894

[16] Yoshida H, Matsui T, Yamamoto A, et al. XBP1 mRNA is induced by ATF6 and spliced by IRE1 in response to ER stress to produce a highly active transcription factor. Cell. 2001;**107**:881-891

[17] Shin BS, Maag D, Roll-Mecak A, et al. Uncoupling of initiation factor eIF5B/IF2 GTPase and translational activities by mutations that lower ribosome affinity. Cell. 2002;**111**:1015-1025

[18] Lu PD, Harding HP, Ron D. Translation reinitiation at alternative open reading frames regulates gene expression in an integrated stress response. The Journal of Cell Biology. 2004;**167**:27-33

[19] Halperin L, Jung J, Michalak M. The many functions of the endoplasmic reticulum chaperones and folding enzymes. IUBMB Life. 2014;**66**:318-326

[20] Novoa I, Zeng H, Harding HP, et al. Feedback inhibition of the unfolded protein response by GADD34-mediated dephosphorylation of eIF2alpha. The Journal of Cell Biology. 2001;**153**:1011-1102

[21] Wang XZ, Ron D. Stress-induced phosphorylation and activation of the transcription factor CHOP (GADD153) by p38 MAP kinase. Science. 1996;**272**:1347-1349

[22] Haas IG, Wabl M. Immunoglobulin heavy chain binding protein. Nature. 1983;**306**:387-389

[23] Munro S, Pelham HR. An Hsp70-like protein in the ER: Identity with the 78 kd glucose-regulated protein and immunoglobulin heavy chain binding protein. Cell. 1986;**46**:291-300

[24] Normington K, Kohno K, Kozutsumi Y, et al. S. cerevisiae encodes an essential protein homologous in sequence and function to mammalian BiP. Cell. 1989;**57**:1223-1236

[25] Pouyssegur J, Shiu RP, Pastan I. Induction of two transformation- sensitive membrane polypeptides in normal fibroblasts by a block in glycoprotein synthesis or glucose deprivation. Cell. 1977;**11**:941-947

[26] Nishitoh H, Matsuzawa A, Tobiume K, et al. HAsk1 is essential for endoplasmic reticulum stress-induced neuronal cell death triggered by expanded polyglutamine repeats. Genes & Development. 2002;**16**:1345-1355

[27] Hetz C, Glimcher LH. Fine-tuning of the unfolded protein response: Assembling the IRE1 alpha interactome. Molecular Cell. 2009;**35**:551-561

[28] Upton JP, Wang L, Han D, et al. Ire1alpha cleaves select microRNAs during ER stress to derepress translation of proapoptotic caspase-2. Science. 2012;**338**:818-822

[29] Xiang C, Wang Y, Zhang H, Han F. The role of endoplasmic reticulum stress in neurodegenerative disease. Apoptosis. 2017;**22**(1):1-26

[30] English AR, Voeltz GK. Endoplasmic reticulum structure and interconnections with other organelles. Cold Spring Harbor Perspectives in Biology. 2013;**5**:a013227

[31] Schwarz DS, Blower MD. The endoplasmic reticulum: Structure, function and response to cellular signaling. Cellular and Molecular Life Sciences. 2016;**73**:79-94

[32] Burgoyne T, Patel S, Eden ER. Calcium signaling at ER membrane contact sites. Biochimica et Biophysica Acta (BBA) - Molecular Cell Research. 2014;**1853**:2012-2017

[33] Xia MF, Zhang YZ, Jin K, Lu ZT, Zeng Z, Xiong W. Communication between mitochondria and other organelles: A brand-new perspective on mitochondria in cancer. Cell & Bioscience. 2019;**9**:1-19

[34] Friedman JR, Lackner LL, West M, DiBenedetto JR, Nunnari J, Voeltz GK. ER tubules mark sites of mitochondrial division. Science. 2011;**334**:358-362

[35] Area-Gomez E, De Groof A, Bonilla E, Montesinos J, Tanji K, Boldogh I, et al. A key role for MAM in mediating mitochondrial dysfunction in Alzheimer disease. Cell Death & Disease. 2018;**9**:1-10

[36] Gómez-Suaga P, Bravo-San Pedro JM, González-Polo RA, Fuentes JM, Niso-Santano M. ER-mitochondria signaling in Parkinson's disease review-article. Cell Death & Disease. 2018;**9**:1-12

[37] Uddin MS, Tewari D, Sharma G, Kabir MT, Barreto GE, Bin-Jumah MN, et al. Molecular mechanisms of ER stress and UPR in the pathogenesis of Alzheimer's disease. Molecular Neurobiology. 2020;**57**:1-18

[38] Carrara M, Prischi F, Nowak PR, Kopp MC, Ali MMU. Noncanonical binding of BiP ATPase domain to Ire1 and Perk is dissociated by unfolded protein CH1 to initiate ER stress signaling. eLife. 2015;**4**:e03522

[39] Hu H, Tian M, Ding C, Yu S. The C/EBP homologous protein (CHOP) transcription factor functions in endoplasmic reticulum stress-induced apoptosis and microbial infection. Frontiers in Immunology. 2019;**10**:1-13

[40] Ron D, Hubbard SR. How IRE1 reacts to ER stress. Cell. 2008;**132**:24-26

[41] Hollien J, Weissman JS. Decay of endoplasmic reticulum-localized mRNAs during the unfolded protein response. Science. 2006;**313**:104-107

[42] Hollien J, Lin JH, Li H, Stevens N, Walter P, Weissman JS. Regulated Ire1-dependent decay of messenger RNAs in mammalian cells. The Journal of Cell Biology. 2009;**186**:323-331

[43] Ghemrawi R, Khair M. Endoplasmic reticulum stress and unfolded protein response in neurodegenerative diseases. International Journal of Molecular Sciences. 2020;**21**(17):6127

[44] Hirtz D, Thurman DJ, Gwinn-Hardy K, Mohamed M, Chaudhuri AR, Zalutsky R. How common are the "common" neurologic disorders? Neurology. 2007;**68**:326-337

[45] Bellucci A, Navarria L, Zaltieri M, Falarti E, Bodei S, Sigala S, et al. Induction of the unfolded protein response by α-synuclein in experimental models of Parkinson's disease. Journal of Neurochemistry. 2011;**116**:588-605

[46] Bellani S, Mescola A, Ronzitti G, Tsushima H, Tilve S, Canale C, et al. GRP78 clustering at the cell surface of neurons transduces the action of exogenous alpha-synuclein. Cell Death and Differentiation. 2014;**21**:1971-1983

[47] Valdés P, Mercado G, Vidal RL, Molina C, Parsons G, Court FA, et al. Control of dopaminergic neuron survival by the unfolded protein response transcription factor XBP1. Proceedings of the National Academy of Sciences of the United States of America. 2014;**111**:6804-6809

[48] Goedert M, Spillantini MG, Del Tredici K, Braak H. 100 years of Lewy pathology. Nature Reviews. Neurology. 2013;**9**:13-24

[49] Witt SN. Molecular chaperones, α-synuclein, and neurodegeneration. Molecular Neurobiology. 2013;**47**:552-560

[50] Malek N, Swallow D, Grosset KA, Anichtchik O, Spillantini M, Grosset DG. Alpha-synuclein in peripheral tissues and body fluids as a biomarker for Parkinson's disease—A systematic review. Acta Neurologica Scandinavica. 2014;**130**:59-72

[51] Santos LE, Ferreira ST. Crosstalk between endoplasmic reticulum stress and brain inflammation in Alzheimer's disease. Neuropharmacology. 2018;**136**:350-360

[52] Lindholm D, Wootz H, Korhonen L. ER stress and neurodegenerative diseases. Cell Death and Differentiation. 2006;**13**:385-392

[53] Mattsson N, Zetterberg H, Janelidze S, Insel PS, Andreasson U, Stomrud E, et al. Plasma tau in Alzheimer disease. Neurology. 2016;**87**:1827-1835

[54] Devi L, Ohno M. PERK mediates eIF2αphosphorylation responsible for BACE1 elevation, CREB dysfunction and neurodegeneration in a mouse model of Alzheimer's disease. Neurobiology of Aging. 2014;**35**:2272-2281

[55] O'Connor T, Sadleir KR, Maus E, Velliquette RA, Zhao J, Cole SL, et al. Phosphorylation of the translation initiation factor eIF2α increases BACE1 levels and promotes Amyloidogenesis. Neuron. 2008;**60**:988-1009

[56] Lee MS, Kim YJ. Signaling pathways downstream of pattern recognition receptors and their cross talk. Annual Review of Biochemistry. 2007;**76**:447-480

[57] Lin JH, Walter P, Yen TSB. Endoplasmic reticulum stress in disease pathogenesis. Annual Review of Pathology. 2008;**3**:399-425

[58] Hotamisligil GS. Role of endoplasmic reticulum stress and c-Jun NH2-terminal kinase pathways in inflammation and origin of obesity and diabetes. Diabetes. 2005;**54**(Suppl. 2):S73-S78

[59] Bailey D, O'Hare P. Transmembrane bZIP transcription factors in ER stress signaling and the unfolded protein response. Antioxidants & Redox Signaling. 2007;**9**:2305-2321

[60] Todd DJ, Lee AH, Glimcher LH. The endoplasmic reticulum stress response in immunity and autoimmunity. Nature Reviews. Immunology. 2008;**8**:663-674

[61] Leitman J, Ulrich Hartl F, Lederkremer GZ. Soluble forms of polyQ-expanded huntingtin rather than large aggregates cause endoplasmic reticulum stress. Nature Communications. 2013;**4**:2753

[62] Duennwald ML, Lindquist S. Impaired ERAD and ER stress are early and specific events in polyglutamine toxicity. Genes & Development. 2008;**22**(23):3308-3319

[63] Yang H, Liu C, Zhong Y, 6Luo S, Monteiro MJ, Fang S. Huntingtin interacts with the cue domain of gp78 and inhibits gp78 binding to ubiquitin and p97/VCP. PLoS One. 2010;**5**(1):e8905

[64] Carnemolla A, Fossale E, Agostoni E, Michelazzi S, Calligaris R, De Maso L, et al. Rrs1 is involved in endoplasmic reticulum stress response in Huntington

disease. The Journal of Biological Chemistry. 2009;**284**(27):18167-18173

[65] Reijonen S, Putkonen N, Norremolle A, Lindholm D, Korhonen L. Inhibition of endoplasmic reticulum stress counteracts neuronal cell death and protein aggregation

[66] Leitman J, Barak B, Benyair R, Shenkman M, Ashery U, Hartl FU, et al. ER stress-induced eIF2-alpha phosphorylation underlies sensitivity of striatal neurons to pathogenic huntingtin. PLoS One. 2014;**9**(3):e90803

Section 2

Cancer Histopathology

Chapter 7

Neoplasia

Flora Thanadar Ajmiree

Abstract

Due to our environmental change, neoplasia is much more common worldwide. And nowadays some well-developed modalities of cancer diagnosis are available. That is why we have to learn about neoplasia. Neoplasia is defined as a genetic disorientation of cell growth that is triggered by acquired or less commonly inherited mutations affecting a single cell and its clonal progeny. Nonlethal genetic damage lies at the heart of carcinogenesis. Genetic damage may be acquired or inherited. Mainly four types of cellular genes are involved in molecular carcinogenesis: 1. Growth-promoting proto-oncogenes, 2. Growth-inhibiting tumor suppressor genes, 3. Genes that regulate apoptosis, and 4. Genes involved in DNA repair. Carcinogenesis is a multistep process. Each cancer must result from accumulation of multiple mutations. Besides this carcinogens like chemicals, microbial and radiation can cause genetic damage or mutations that initiate cancer. Initiation of carcinogenesis is started with mutations and promotion of tumor growth is in involved cell. Due to the advanced tumor diagnosis, it helps in early tumor detection. We can identify a malignant cell by cell criteria. This property helps us to treat cancer early and help us to cure it. Therefore, nowadays tumor pathology or neoplasia is a topic of the time.

Keywords: neoplasia, definition, classifications, epidemiology of cancer, molecular basis of cancer, Warburg effect, invasion and metastasis, chemical and radiation carcinogenesis, microbial carcinogenesis, lab diagnosis, tumor marker, paraneoplastic syndrome, tumor staging

1. Introduction

Neoplasia → new growth

Oncology → study of tumors or neoplasm.

('Oncos' means Tumor)

Definition → Neoplasia is defined as a genetic disorientation of cell growth that is triggered by acquired or less commonly inherited mutations affecting a single cell or its clonal progeny [1].

These mutations give the neoplastic cells a survival and growth advantage, resulting in excessive proliferation that is independent of physiological growth signals and control.

1.1 Salient features of neoplasia

- **Origin:** Neoplasms arise from cells that normally maintain a proliferative capacity.

- **Genetic disorder:** Cancer is due to permanent genetic changes in the cell, known as mutations. These mutations may occur in genes that regulate cell growth, apoptosis, or DNA repair.
- **Heritable:** The genetic alterations are passed down to the daughter tumor cells.
- **Monoclonal:** All the neoplastic cells within an individual tumor originate from a single cell or clone of cells that have undergone a genetic change. Thus, tumors are said to be monoclonal.
- **Carcinogenic stimulus:** The stimulus responsible for the uncontrolled cell proliferation may not be identified or is not known.
- **Autonomy:** In neoplasia, there is excessive and unregulated proliferation of cells that do not obey the normal regulatory control. The cell proliferation is independent of physiologic growth stimuli. But tumors are dependent on the host for their nutrition and blood supply.
- **Irreversible:** Neoplasm is irreversible and persists even after the inciting stimulus is withdrawn or gone.
- **Differentiation:** It refers to the extent to which the tumor cells resemble the cell of origin.
- A tumor may show varying degrees of differentiation ranging from relatively mature structures that mimic normal tissues (well-differentiated) to cells, so primitive that the the cell of origin cannot be identified (poorly differentiated).
- **Oncology: Study of neoplasms** [1].

1.2 Six P's of neoplasm

- Purposeless.
- Progressive.
- Proliferation unregulated.
- Preys on host.
- Persists even after withdrawal of stimulus (autonomous).
- Permanent genetic change in the cell.

1.3 Components of neoplasms

Tumors (both benign and malignant) consist of two basic components:
Microscopic:

1. **Parenchyma:** It is made up of neoplastic cells. The nomenclature and biological behavior of tumors are based primarily on the parenchymal component of tumor.

2. **Stroma:** It is the supporting, nonneoplastic tissue derived from the host.

    - **Components:** Connective tissue, blood vessels, and inflammatory cells (e.g., macrophages and lymphocytes).

    - **Inflammatory reaction:** Stroma may show inflammatory reactions in and around the tumors. It may be due to ulceration and secondary infection in the tumors, especially on the surface of the body.

      This type of inflammatory reaction may be acute, chronic, or rarely granulomatous reaction. Some tumors show inflammatory reactions even in the absence of ulceration. It is due to cell-mediated immunologic response of the host against the tumor in an attempt to destroy the tumor. For example, lymphocytes in the stroma are seen in seminoma testis and medullary carcinoma of the breast.

3. **Importance of stroma:** It is required for growth, survival, and replication of tumor (through blood supply) cells [1].

4. **Tumor consistency depends on amount of stroma:**

    - **Soft and fleshy:** These tumors have scanty stroma.

    - **Desmoplasia:** Parenchymal tumor cells may stimulate the formation of an abundant collagenous stroma.

    - referred to as desmoplasia. For example, some carcinomas in female breasts have stony hard consistency (or scirrhous) [1].

2. Classification

Tumors are classified as benign and malignant, depending on the biological behavior of a tumor.

1. **Benign tumors:** They have relatively innocent microscopic and gross characteristics

    - Remain localized without invasion or metastasis.

    - Well-differentiated: Their cells closely resemble their tissue of origin.

    - Prognosis: It is very good, can be cured by surgical removal in most patients and the patient generally survives [1].

2. **Malignant tumors:** Cancer is the general term used for malignant tumors. The term "cancer" is derived from the Latin word for crab, because similar to a crab, malignant tumors adhere to any part that they seize on, in an obstinate manner.

    - Invasion: Malignant tumors invade or infiltrate into the adjacent tissues or structures.

- Metastasis: Cancers spread to distant sites metastasize), where the malignant cells reside, grow, and again invade.

- Exception: Basal cell carcinoma of the skin, which is histologically malignant (i.e., it invades aggressively), rarely metastasizes to distant sites. Glioma is a malignant tumor of CNS.

- Prognosis: Most malignant tumors cause death [1].

2.1 Benign tumors

- Remain localized at their site of origin.
- Generally amenable to surgical removal.
- Suffix → Oma follows the name of the cell type from which tumor arises.
- In complaints of benign mesenchymal tumors.
- Tumors from fibrous tissue → Fibroma
- Tumors from cartilaginous tissue → Chondroma
- Benign epithelial tumors with complex nomenclature.
- Depending on cell of origin.
- From glandular stromal origin-Adenomas, for example, tumors from renal tubular cell
- May not be from glandular stromal origin, for example, tumor from adrenal cortex.
- Depending on macroscopic appearance
- Visible projection above mucosal surface of gastrointestinal tract-polyp
- If there is glandular component present in a polyp it is called –Adenomatous polyp
- Depending on microscopic pattern:
- Microscopic finger-like projection from epithelial surface –*Papillomas*
- Large cystic masses in ovary—Cystadenoma
- If papillary stromal projection in the cyst is called –*Papillary cystadenomas* [1].

2.2 Malignant tumors

According cancers derived from Latin word for crab.

Tissue of origin	Benign	Malignant
	Composed of one parenchymal cell type	
	Tumors of mesenchymal	
Connective tissue and derivatives	Fibroma lipoma chondroma osteoma	Fibrosarcoma liposarcoma chondrosarcoma osteogenic sarcoma
	Vessels and surface coverings	
Blood vessels	Hemangionma	Angiosarcoma
Lymph vessels	Lymphangioma	Lymphangiosarcoma
Mesothelium	Benign fibrous tumor	Mesothelioma
Brain coverings	Meningioma	Invasive meningioma
	Blood cells and related cells	
Hematopoietic cells		Leukemias
Lymphoid tissue		Lymphomas
	Muscle	
Smooth	Leiomyoma	Leiomyosarcoma
Striated	Rhabdomyoma	Rhabdomyosarcoma
	Tumors of epithelial origin	
Stratified squamous	Squamous cell papilloma	Squamous cell carcinoma
Basal cells of skin or adnexa		Basal cell carcinoma
Epithelial lining of glands or ducts	Adenoma papilloma cystadenoma	Adenocarcinoma papillary carcinomas cystadenoma
Respiratory passages	Bronchial adenoma	Bronchogenic carcinoma
Renal epithelium	Renal tubular adenoma	Renal cell carcinoma
Liver cells	Hepatic adenoma	Hepatocellular carcinoma
URinary tract epithelium (transitional)	Transitional cell papilloma	Transitional cell carcinoma
Placental epithelium	Hydatidiform mole	Choriocatcinoma
Tumors of melanocytes	Nevus	Malignant melanoma
More than one neoplastic cell type tumors, usually derived from one germ cell layer		
Salivary glands	Pleomorphic adenoma (mixed tumor of salivary origin)	Malignant mixed tumor of salivary gland origin
Renal anlage		Wilms tumor
More than one neoplastic cell type derived from more than one germ cell layer—teralogenous		
Totipotent cells in gonads or in embryonic rests	Mature teratoma, dermoid cyst	Immature teratoma, teratocarcinoma

Table 1.
Nomenclature of tumors.

- Can invade and destroy adjacent structures and spread to distant sites → metastasize.
- Sometimes cancers are identified in accordance to their tissue or organ of origin where the organ or tissue of origin is added to descriptors.
- For example Bronchogenic squamous cell carcinoma and renal cell adenocarcinoma.
- In 2% of cases, cell of origin is not known > undifferentiated malignant tumor > mixed tumor.
- Tumors of more than one line of differentiation
- Derived from one germ layer. (Most fall in this group), for example, Mixed tumor of salivary gland.
- Derived from more than one germ layer. e.g. Teratoma contains epithelium, bone, muscle, fat, and nerve (**Tables 1** and **2**) [1].

3. Epidemiology of cancer

1. Global impact of cancer.
2. Environmental factors.
3. Age.
4. Acquired predisposing conditions.
5. Genetic predisposing and interactions between environmental and inherited factors.

Characteristics	**Benign**	**Malignant**
Differentiation/ anaplasia	Well differentiated; structure sometimes typical of tissue of origin	Some lack of differentiation (anaplasia); structure often atypical
Rate of growth	Usually progressive and slow; may come to a standstill or regress; mitotic figures rare and normal	Erratic, may be slow to rapid; mitotic figures may be numerous and abnormal
Local invasion	Usually cohesive, expansile, well-demarcated masses that do not invade or infiltrate surrounding normal tissues	Locally invasive, infiltrating surrounding tissue; sometimes may be misleadingly cohesive and expansile
Metastasis	Absent	Frequent; more likely with large undifferentiated primary tumors

Table 2.
Comparisons between benign and malignant tumors.

3.1 Global impact of cancer

2018 → 9.5 million deaths were caused by cancer worldwide, one in six deaths.

No of cancer cause	No of cancer related deaths
↓	↓
Increase to 21.4 million	Increase to 13.2 million

M/C cancer in men → prostate, lung, colon, rectum.
M/C cancer in women → breast, lung, colon/rectum.
Environmental factors although both genetic and environmental factors contribute, Environmental influences are the dominant risk factors for most cancers. Incidence of cancer increases with age due to according of somatic mutations and decrease in immune competence in older individual [2–5].

3.2 Age

Age was an important implication of the risk of cancer.
Most carcinomas occur in adults older than 55 years of age.
Mean age range for cancer in women – 40 to 79 years and in men – 60 to 79 years.

3.3 Infectious agents

- 15% cancers worldwide are caused directly/indirectly by infectious agents.
- Risk is three times higher in developing countries.

  E.g. Role of HPV → Cervical Carcinoma, Head and neck carcinoma.

3.4 Smoking

- Implicated in cancers of the mouth, larynx, Pharynx, esophagus, Pancreas, bladder, and lung cancers (90%).

3.5 Alcohol consumption

- Increased risk of carcinoma of oropharynx (excluding lip); larynx and esophagus.
- Increases risk of cirrhosis and hepatocellular carcinoma.

  (2) + (3) ace synergistically.

3.6 Diet

- Diet Plays important role in cancers of prostate breast and colorectal cancer.

3.7 Obesity

- Associated with increased cancer risk 14% cancer death in men and 20% cancer death in women. [Risk Associated with obesity]

3.8 Reproductive history

- Lifelong exposure of estrogen increase risk (unopposed by progesterone) of carcinoma of tissue exposed to the hormones. For example-carcinoma of breast and endometrium.

3.9 Environmental carcinogens

For example, U-V- rays from sun, well water (Arsenic) medications (Methotrexate) work place (Asbestos) Home (Grilled meat; High-fat diet, alcohol) (**Table 3**) [2–5].

3.10 Precancerous conditions

- Certain non-neoplastic disorders have association with cancer, termed precancerous conditions.

  They are important to recognize because some precursor lesions can be detected by screening procedures, thereby reducing the risk of developing cancer.

  Examples:

- Skin: Solar actinic keratosis, Marjolin ulcer, Dysplastic nevi, Leukoplakia, Radio dermatitis.
- Oral cavity: Leukoplakia of the oral cavity.
- Female genital tract: Cervical dysplasia, leukoplakia of vulva, endometrial hyperplasia.
- Breast: Intra ductal hyperplasia.
- Esophagus: Barrett's esophagus.
- Stomach: Chronic atrophic gastritis, pernicious anemia.
- Colon: Familial adenomatous polyposis colon.
- Penis: Leukoplakia of penis.
- Lungs: Squamous metaplasia [2–5].

4. Molecular basis of cancer

All cancers display eight fundamental changes in cell physiology, which are considered the hallmarks of cancer.

Pathologic condition	Associated neoplasm(s)	Etiologic agent
Asbestosis, silicosis	Mesothelioma, lung carcinoma	Asbestos fibers, silica particles
Inflammatory bowel disease	Colorectal carcinoma	
Lichen sclerosis	Vulvar squamous cell carcinoma	
Pancreatitis	Pancreatic carcinoma	Alcoholism, germline mutations (e.g., in the trypsinogen gene)
Chronic cholecystitis	Gallbladder cancer	Bile acids, bacteria, gallbladder stones
Reflux esophagitis, Barrett esophagus	Esophageal carcinoma	Gastric acid
Sjogren syndrome, Hashimoto thyroiditis	MALT lymphoma	
Opisthorchis, cholangitis	Cholangiocarcinoma, colon carcinoma	Liver flukes (Opisthorchis viverrinl)
Gastritis/ulcers	Gastric adenocarcinoma, MALT lymphoma	Helicobacter pylori
Hepatitis	Hepatocellular carcinoma	Hepatitis B and/or C virus
Osteomyelitis	Carcinoma in draining sinuses	Bacterial infection
Chronic cervicitis	Cervical carcinoma	Human papillomavirus
Chronic cystitis	Bladder carcinoma	Schistosomiasis

Table 3.
Chronic inflammatory states and cancer.

These changes are:

1. Self-sufficiency in growth signals: Tumors have the capacity to proliferate without external stimuli, usually as a consequence of oncogene activation.

2. Insensitivity to growth-inhibitory signals: Tumors may not respond to molecules that are inhibitory to the proliferation of normal cells such as cyclin-dependent kinases (CDKIs).

3. Altered cellular metabolism: Tumor cells undergo a metabolic switch to aerobic glycolysis, which enables the synthesis of the macromolecules and organelles that are needed for rapid cell growth – called the Warburg effect.

4. Evasion of apoptosis: Tumors are resistant to programmed cell death.

5. Limitless replicative potential (immortality): Tumors have unrestricted proliferative capacity to avoid cellular senescence.

6. Sustained angiogenesis: Tumor cells are not able to grow without vascular supply to bring nutrients, oxygen and remove waste products. So, tumors must induce angiogenesis.

7. Ability to invade and metastasize: Tumor metastases are the cause of the vast majority of cancer deaths [6].

8. Ability to evade the host immune response – cancer cells exhibit a number of alterations (in the innate and adaptive immune system) that allow them to evade the immune response.

   - Protooncogenes: Proto oncogenes have multiple roles but all participate at some level in signaling pathways that drive proliferation.
     - Normal cellular genes, whose products promote cell proliferation.
     - Unmutated version.
     - Proto-oncogenes may encode growth factors, growth factor receptors, signal transducers, transcription factors, or cell cycle components (**Table 4**).
   - Oncogenes:
     - Genes that promote autonomous cell growth in cancer cells are called oncogenes.
     - Mutant versions of proto-oncogenes.
     - Encode proteins called oncoproteins.
     - Have the ability to promote cell growth in the absence of normal growth promoting signal (**Table 5**) [7–10].
   - Tumor suppressor gene:
     - Genes negatively regulate proliferation. Apply brakes or arrest cell cycle to cell proliferation.
     - Abnormalities in these genes lead to failure of growth inhibition.
     - Effect on the regulation of the cell cycle on promote apoptosis, and sometimes do both.
     - Mutation in tumor suppressor gene causes unregulated cell growth.
     - First tumor-suppressor protein discovered was the Retinoblastoma protein (pRb) in retinoblastoma (**Table 6**) [11–14].

5. Altered cellular metabolism in canter cells (Warburg effect)

Cancer cells have different needs than their normal counterpart. Their proliferative rate generally exceeds that of normal cells. Cancer cells must quickly synthesize the structural components (e.g., protein, lipid, etc.) that are required for rapid cell growth (that is to sustain their mitotic activity).

With adequate oxygen supply, cancer cells undergo a metabolic switch to aerobic glycolysis. They develop a distinctive form of cellular metabolism characterized by

Category	Prolo-onicogene	Mode of activation in tumor	Associated human tumor
Growth factors			
PDGFB chain	PDGFB	Overexpression	Astrocytoma
Fibroblast growth factors	HST1	Overexpression	Osteosarcoma stomach cancer bladder
	FGF3	Amplification	Cancer breast cancer melanoma
TGF-a	TGFA	Overexpression	Astrocytomas
HGF	HGF	Overexpression	Hepatocellular carcionmas, thyroid cancer
Growth factor receptors			
EGF-receptor family	ERBB1 (EGFR)	Mutation amplification	Adenocarinoma of lung
	ERBB2 (EGFR)		Breast carcinoma
FMS-like tyrosin kinase 3	FLT3	Point mutation	Leukemia
Receptor for neurotrophic factors	RET	Point mutation	Multiple endocrine neoplasia 2A and B, familial medullary thyroid carcinomas
PDGF receptor	PDGFRB	Overexpression, translocation	Gliomas, leukemias
Receptor for KIT ligand	KIT	Point mutation	Gastrointeslinal stromal tumors, seminomas, leukemias
ALK receptor	ALK	Translocation, fusion gene formation point mutaion	Adenocarcinoma of lunk, certain lymphomas neuroblastoma
Proteins involved in signal transduction			
GTP-binding (G) prodeins	KRAS	Point mutation	Colon, lung, and pancreatic tumors
	HRAS	Point mutation	Bladder and kidney tumors
	NRAS	Point mutation	Melanomas, hematologic malignancies, Uveal melanoma
	GNAQ	Point mutation	Pituitary adenoma, other endocrine tumors
	GNAS	Point mutation	
Nonreceptor tyrosin kinase	ABL	Translocation point mutation	Chronic myelogenous leukemia
			Acute lymphoblastic, leukemia
RAS signal transtiuction	BRAF	Point mutation, Translocation	Melanomas, leukemias, colon carcinoma, other
Notch signal transduction	NOTCH1	Point mutation, translocation gene reanangement	Leukemias, lymphomas, breast carcinoma
JAK/STAT signal transduction	JAK2	Translocation	Myeloproliferative disorders acute lymphoblastic leukemia

Category	Prolo-onicogene	Mode of activation in tumor	Associated human tumor
Nuclear Regulatory proteins			
Transcriptional activators	MYC	Translocation	Burkitt lymphoma
	NMYC	Amplification	Neuroblastoma
Cell cycle regulators			
Cyclins	CCND1 (Cyclin D1)	Translocation	Mantle cell lymphoma, multiple myeloma
		Amplification	Breast and esophageal cancers
Cyclin-dependent kinase	CDK4	Amplification or point mutation	Glioblastoma, melanoma, sarcoma

Table 4.
Selected oncogenes, their mode of activation, and associated human tumors.

Cell cycle component	Main function
Cyclins and cyclin-dependent kinases	
CDK4; D cyclins	Form a complex that phosporylates RB, allowing the cell to progress througe the G, regtriction point
Cell cycle inhibitors	
CIP/KIP family: p21, p27 (CDKN1A-D)	Block the cell cycle by binding to cyclin-CDK complexes
	p21 Is induced by the tumor suppressor p53
	p27 responds to growth suppressors such as TGF-B
INK4/ARF familly (CDKN2A-C)	p16/ink4A and promotes the inhibitory effects of RB
	p14ARF increases p53 levels by inhibiting MDM2 activity
Cell cycle checkpoint components	
RB	Tumor suppressive “pocket” protein that binds E2F transcription factors in its hypophosphorylated state, preventing G,/S transition; also interacts with several transcription factors that regulate differentiation
p53	Tumor suppressor altered in the majority of cancers; causes cell cycle arrest and apoptosis. Acts mainly through p21 to cause cell cycle arrest. Causes apoptosis by inducing the transcription of pro-apoptotic genes such as BAX. Levels of p53 are negatively regulated by MDM2 through a feedback loop. p53 is required for the G1/S checkpoint and is a main component of the G2/M checkpoint.

Table 5.
Cell cycle components and inhibitors that are frequently mutated in cancer.

increased amount of glucose uptake and increased conversion of glucose to lactose (fermentation) via the glycolytic pathway. This aerobic glycolysis is called the Warburg effect. It was described in 1930 by Otto Warburg and is not cancer-specific but observed in growing cells and it becomes “fixed” in cancer cells. It is seen because tumor cells have M2 isoform of pyruvate kinase enzyme.

Aerobic glycolysis provides metabolic intermediates that are needed for the synthesis of cellular components in rapidly dividing tumor cells. This cannot be met with normal mitochondrial oxidative phosphorylation.

Gene	Protein	Function	Familial syndromes	Sporadic cancers
Inhibitors of mitogenic signaling pathways				
APC	Adenomatous polyposis coli protein	Inhibitor of WNT signating	Familial colonic polyps and carcinomas	Carcinomas of stomach, colon, pancreas; melanoma
NF1	Neurofibromin-1	Inhibitor of RAS/MAPK signaling	Neurofibromatosis type 1 (neurofibromas and malignant peripheral nerve	Neuroblastoma, juvenile myeloid leukemia sheath tumors)
NF2	Merlin	Cytosketetal stability, hippo pathway signaling	Neurolibromatosis type 2 (acoustic schwannoma and meningioma)	Schwannoma, meningioma
PTCH	Patched	Inhibitor of Hedgehog signaling	Gorlin syndrome (basal cell carcinoma, medulioblastoma, several benign tumors)	Basal cell carcinoma, medulioblastoma
PTEN	Phosphatase and tensin homologue	Inhibitor of pi3k/AKT signaling	Cowden syndrome (variety of benign skin, g1, and CNS growths; breast, endometrial, and thyroid carcinoma)	Diverse cancers, particularly carcinomas and lymphoid tumors
SMAD2, SMAD4	SMAD2, SMAD4	Component of the TGFB signaling pathway, repressors of MYC and CDK4 expression, inducers of CDK inhibitor expression	Juvenile polyposis	Frequenthy mutated (along with other components of the TGFB signaling pathway) in colonic and pancreatic carcinoma
Inhibltors of cell cycle progression				
RB	Retinoblastoma (RB) protein	Inhibitor of G1/S transition during cell cycle progression	Familial retinoblastoma syndrome (retinoblastoma, osteosarcoma, other sarcomas)	retinoblastoma; osteosarcoma carcinomas of breast, colon, lung
CDKN2A	p16/INK43 and p14/ARF	p16; Negative regulator of cyclin-dependent kinases; p14, indirect activator of p53	Familial melanoma	Pancreatic, breast, and esophageal carcinoma, melanoma, certain leukemias
Inhibitors of pro-growth' programs of metabolism and angiogenesis				
VHL	Von hippel lindsu (VHL) protein	Inhibitor of hypoxia-induced transcription factors (e.g, HF1a)	Von Hippel lindau syndrome (cerebellar hemangioblastoma, retinal angioma, renal cell carcinoma)	Renal cell carcinoma
STK11	Liver Kinase B1 (LKB1) or STK11	Activator of AMPK family of kinases; suppresses cell growth when cell nutrient and energy levels are low	Peutz-Jeghers syndrome (G1polyps, G1 cancers, pancreatic carcinoma and other carcinomas)	Diverse carcinomas (5%-20% of cases, depending on type)

Gene	Protein	Function	Familial syndromes	Sporadic cancers
SDHB, SDHD	Succinate dehydrogenase complex subunits B and D	TCA cycle, oxidative phosphorylation	Familial paraganglioma, familial pheochromocytoma	Paraganglioma
Inhibitors of genomic Stability				
CDH1	E-cadherin	cell adhesion, inhibition of cell mobity	Familial gastric cancer	Gastric carcinoma, lobular breast carcinoma
Enablers of genomic stability				
TP53	p53 protein	Cell cycle arrest and apoptosis in response to DNA damage	LI-Fraumeni syndrome (diverse cancers)	Most human cancers
DNA repair factors				
BRCA1, BRCA2	Breast cancer-1 and breast cancer-2 (BRCA1 and BRCA2)	Repair of double-stranded breaks in DNA	Familial breast and ovarian carcinoma; carcinomas of male breast; chronic lymphocytic leukemia (BRCA2)	Rare
MSH2, MLH1, MSH6	MSH1, MLH1, MSH6	DNA mismatch repair	Hereditaty nonpolyposis colon carcinoma	Colonic and endometrial carcinoma
Uniknown mechanlams				
WT1	Wilms tumor-1 (WT1)	Transcription factor	Familial Wilms tumor	Wilms tumor, certain leukemias
MEN1	Menin	Transcription factor	Multiple endocrine neoplasia-1 (MEN1; pituitary, parathyroid, and pancreatic endocrine tumors)	Pituitary, parathyroid, and pancreatic endocrine tumors

Table 6.
Selected tumor suppressor genes and associated familal syndromes and cencer. Sorted by Cancer Hallmarks.

Clinical utility: The "glucose-hunger" of tumors is made for visualization of tumors in positron emission tomography (PET) scanning. In PET scanning, patients are injected with 18F-fluorodeoxyglucose (a8-FDG- a non-metabolizable derivative of glucose) which is preferentially taken up into tumor cells (and also actively dividing normal cells, for example., bone marrow cells). Most tumors are PET-positive, and markedly positive are the rapidly growing tumors [15].

6. Invasion and metastasis

6.1 Locally malignant tumor

Definition: The malignant tumors that are locally invasive but show little or no tendency to metastasize are called locally malignant tumors.

- Examples:

    1. Basal cell carcinoma of skin.

    2. Glioma/glial cell carcinoma of central nervous system.

    3. Giant cell tumor of bone.

    4. Ameloblastoma.

    5. Craniopharyngioma.

- Local Invasion:

    A. Benign tumor:

    - Grow as cohesive expansile masses.

    - Remain localized to their site of origin.

    - Do not have the capacity to infiltrate, invade, or metastasize to distant sites.

    - Sometimes they develop a fibrous capsule.

    B. Malignant Tumor:

    - Invasive and can be expected to penetrate the wall.

    - Such invasiveness makes their surgical resection difficult.

Mechanism of tumor invasion:

It involves following steps:

1. Detachment ("loosening up") of the tumor cells from each other

    - Tumor cells remain attached to each other by several adhesion molecules, such as cadherins.

    - In several carcinomas, including adenocarcinoma.

2. Degradation of extracellular matrix

    By elaborating protease enzymes-matrix metalloproteinases (MMPs), cathepsin D, and urokinase plasminogen activator.

3. Attachment to novel extracellular matrix components: Tumor cells bind to laminin and fibronectin via cell surface receptors.

4. Migration of tumor cells:

- It is the final step of invasion, propelling tumor cells through the degraded basement membranes and zones of matrix proteolysis.
- Stimulated and directed by tumor cell-derived cytokines, such as autocrine motility factors [16, 17].

6.2 Metastasis

Definition: Metastasis is defined by the spread of a tumor to sites that are physically discontinuous with the primary tumor. Or, tumor implant away from primary site to a distant place, without any communication with primary site, is known as metastasis.

- Benign tumor: do not metastasize.
- Malignant tumor: few exceptions, all cancers can metastasize.
- The most common sites of cancer metastasis are the lungs, liver, bones, and brain.
- Although most cancers have the ability to spread in many different parts of the body.
- Exception: Locally invasive cancer. Approximately 30% of newly diagnosed solid tumors (excluding skin cancers other than melanomas) present with metastases.
- Metastatic spread strongly reduces the possibility of cure.

6.3 Pathways of spread

1. Direct seeding of body cavities or surfaces,
2. Lymphatic spread, and
3. Hematogenous spread.

6.4 Direct seeding of body cavities or surfaces

Most often involved is the peritoneal cavity, but any other cavity—pleural, pericardial, subarachnoid, and joint space—may be affected.

- Example: In the female, gastric carcinoma may metastasize through peritoneal cavity to one or both ovaries producing secondary tumors termed krukenberg tumors.
- Sometimes mucus-secreting appendiceal carcinomas or ovarian carcinomas fill the peritoneal cavity with a gelatinous neoplastic mass referred to as pseudomyxoma peritonei.

DOI: http://dx.doi.org/10.5772/intechopen.109512

6.5 Lymphatic spread

- Transport through lymphatics is the most common pathway for the initial dissemination of carcinomas but sarcomas may also use this route.

- Examples: a. Carcinomas of the upper outer quadrant of the breast usually spread first to axillary lymph nodes and those of the inner quadrants to the nodes along the internal mammary arteries then the infra-clavicular and supraclavicular may become involved.

- Bronchogenic carcinoma first metastasizes first to the hilar and mediastinal lymph nodes.

6.6 Hematogenous spread

Hematogenous spread is typical of large masses but is also seen with carcinomas.

- Because ultimately there are numerous interconnections between the vascular and the lymphatic systems.

- Arteries are less (due to thicker wall) easily penetrated than veins.

Sentinel lymph node:
Definition: A "sentinel lymph node" is the first regional lymph node that reaches lymph flow from a primary tumor.

- Sentinel node mapping can be done by injection of radio-labeled tracers or colored dyes.

- Biopsy of sentinel nodes is often used to assess the presence or absence of metastatic lesions in the lymph nodes.

- Examples: In breast cancer, determining the involvement of axillary lymph nodes is important for assessing the future course of the disease and for selecting suitable therapeutic strategies.

- Skip metastasis:

- Usually cancers metastasize along the natural lymphatic drainage of that tissue.

- However local lymph node may be bypassed, which is known as skip metastasis.

- Cause:

    1. Lymphangitis.

    2. Radiation.

    3. Surgical intervention.

    4. Developmental anomalies.

6.7 Mechanism of metastasis of malignant tumor

- Metastasis is a multistep process that allows tumor cells to move from one site to another.
- These steps include:

  1. Detachment of invasive cells from the main tumor mass.
  2. Invasion of the basement membrane and the connective tissue.
  3. Intravasation (i.e., entry of tumor cells into the vessel).
  4. Dissemination of tumor cells in the intravascular fluid (blood or lymph).
  5. Anchorage (i.e., attachment of tumor cells to endothelial cells at a distant site).
  6. Extravasation (i.e., emigration of tumor cells through the vessel wall).
  7. Proliferation at the distant site [16, 17].

6.8 Autophagy and evasion of immune surveillance

6.8.1 Autophagy

Autophagy ("self- eating") is the process in which lysosomal enzymes digest the own components of the cell during stress. It is a survival mechanism that occurs during a state of severe nutrient deficiency. By this mechanism, the starved cell can live by eating its own contents (e.g., organelles, proteins, and membranes) and by recycling these contents to provide nutrients and energy.

If this adaptive mechanism fails, the cells die.

Autophagy in cancer: Role of autophagy in the development and progression of cancer is complex and represents a double-edged sword. Several autophagy genes (e.g., Beclin-1 and some Atg genes) that promote autophagy, act as tumor suppressors and are deleted or mutated in many cancers. Tumor cells may accumulate mutations that deranges the pathways that induce autophagy and allows the cancer cells to grow without triggering autophagy. Tumor cells may corrupt the autophagy process to provide nutrients for continued growth and survival. On the other hand, autophagy can protect cancer cells if they are deprived of nutrients or oxygen because of therapy or insufficient blood supply [18, 19].

6.8.2 Several mechanisms may be operative by which tumor cells escape or evade the immune system:

- Selective outgrowth of antigen-negative variants: During tumor progression, strongly immunogenic subclones may be eliminated.
- Loss or reduced expression of MHC molecules: Tumor cells may fail to express normal levels of HLA class I molecules, thereby escaping attack by cytotoxic T cells. Such cells, however, may trigger NK cells.

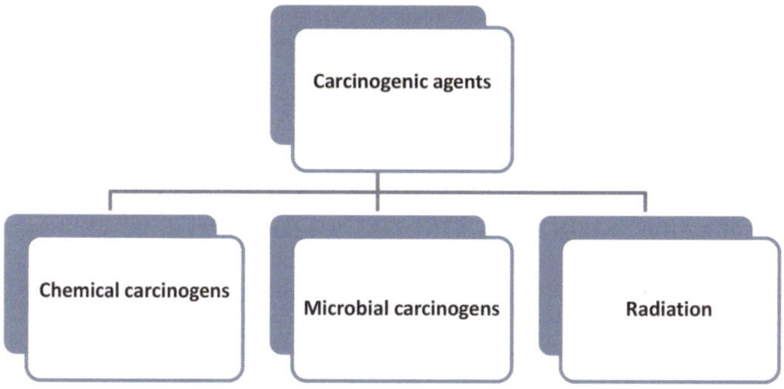

Figure 1.
Major types of carcinogenic agents.

- Lack of co-stimulation: Sensitization of T cells requires two signals, one by a foreign peptide presented by MHC molecules and the other by co-stimulatory molecules. Although tumor cells may express peptide antigens with class I molecules, they often do not express co-stimulatory molecules.

- Immunosuppression: Many oncogenic agents (e.g., chemicals and ionizing radiation) suppress host immune responses.

- Antigen masking: The cell surface antigens of tumors may be hidden, or masked, from the immune system by glycocalyx molecules, such as sialic acid-containing mucopolysaccharides.

- Apoptosis of cytotoxic T cells: Some melanomas and hepatocellular carcinomas express FasL which kills T lymphocytes that come in contact with tumor cells (**Figure 1**) [20].

7. Chemical and radiation carcinogenesis

7.1 Chemical carcinogenesis

Sir Percival Pott (London surgeon) first related scrotum skin cancer in the chimney sweeps to a specific chronic chemical exposure to soot. Based on this, a rule was made that chimney sweep members must bathe daily and this public health measure controlled scrotal skin cancer. Japanese investigators (Yamagiva and Ichikawa) experimentally produced skin cancers in rabbits by using coal tar. Subsequently, hundreds of chemical carcinogens were discovered (**Table** 7).

7.2 Direct-acting agents

Direct-acting chemical agents do not require metabolic conversion to become carcinogenic, but most of them are weak carcinogens. Some of the drugs (e.g., alkylating agents) are used to cure, control, or delay recurrence of some cancer (e.g., leukemia, lymphoma) and may produce a second form of cancer (e.g., acute myeloid leukemia) later.

7.3 Alkylating agents

- Source: many cancer chemotherapeutic drugs (e.g. Cyclophosphamide, cisplatin, and busulfan) are alkylating agents.

Direct-acting carcinogens
Alkylating agents
B-Propiolactone
Dimethyl sulfate
Diepoxybutane
Anticancer drugs (cyclophosphamide, chlorambucil, nitrosoureas, and other)
Acylating agents
1-acetyl-imidazole
Dimethylcarbamyl chloride
Procarcinogens that require metabolic activation
Polycyclic and heterocyclic aromatic hydrocarbons
Benz[a] anthracene
Benzo[a] pyrene
Dibenz[a,h]anthracene
3-Methylcholanthrene
7,12-Dimethylbenz[a]anthracene
Aromatic amines, amides, azo dyes
2-Naphthylamine (B-naphthylamine)
Benzidine
2-Acetylaminofluorene
Dimethylaminoazobenzene (Butter yellow)
Natural plant and microblal products
Aflatoxin B,
Griseofulvin
Cycasin
Safrole
Betel nuts
Others
Nitrosamine and amldes
Vinyl chloride, nickel, chromium
Insecticides, funglcides
Polychlorinated blphenyls

Table 7.
Major chemical carcinogens.

- Mechanism of action: alkylating agents contain electron-deficient atoms that react with electron-rich atoms in DNA. These drugs not only destroy cancer cells by damaging DNA but also injure normal cells.

- Cancers produced: Solid and hematological malignancies (**Table 8** and **Figure 2**) [21, 22].

7.4 Radiation carcinogenesis

Radiation is a well-known carcinogen.

Latency: Extremely long latent period is common and It has a cumulative effect. Radiation has also additive or synergistic effects with other potential carcinogenic agents.

Types of radiation: They are divided into two types, namely:

1. Ultraviolet (UV) rays of sunlight, and

2. Ionizing electromagnetic and particulate radiation.

Ultraviolet rays:-.

They are derived from the sunlight.

Tumors caused: Skin cancer, namely.

1. Squamous cell carcinoma,

2. Basal cell carcinoma, and

3. Malignant melanoma.

They are more common on parts of the body regularly exposed to sunlight and ultraviolet light (UVL).

Risk factors.

The amount of damage incurred depends on:

- Type of UV rays.

    - Intensity of exposure.

    - Protective mantle of melanin.

    - Melanin absorbs UV radiation and has a protective effect.

    - Skin cancers are more common in fair-skinned people and those living in a geographic location receiving a greater amount of sunlight (e.g., Queensland, Australia, close to the equator).

Pathogenesis.

- UV radiation leads to formation of pyrimidine dimers in DNA, which is a type of DNA damage that is responsible for carcinogenicity.

Agents or groups of agents	Human cancers for which reasonable evidence is available	Typical use or occurrence
Arsenic and arsenic compounds	Lung carcinoma, skin carcinoma	By-product of metal smelting; component of alloys, electrical and semiconductor devices, medications and herbicides, fungicides, and animal dips
Asbestos	Lung, esophageal, gastric, and colon carcinoma; mesothelioma	Formerly used for many applications because of fire, heat, and friction resistance; still found in existing construction as well as fire-resistant textiles, friction materials (i.e., brake linings), underlayment and roofing papers, and floor tiles
Benzene	Acute myeloid leukemia	Principal component of light oil; despite known risk, many applications exist in printing and lithography, paint, rubber, dry cleaning, adhesives and coatings, and detergents; formerly widely used as solvent and fumigant
Beryllium and beryllium compounds	Lung carcinoma	Missile fuel and space vehicles; hardener for lightweight metal alloys, particularly in aerospace applications and nuclear reactors
Cadmlum and cadmium compounds	Prostate carcinoma	Uses include yellow pigments and phosphors; found in solders; used in batteries and as alloy and in metal platings and coatings
Chromium compounds	Lung carcinoma	Component of metal alloys, paints, pigments, and preservatives
Nickel compounds	Lung and oropharyngeal carcinoma	Nickel plating; component of ferrous alloys, ceramics, and batteries; by-product of stainless-steel arc welding
Radon and its decay products	Lung carcinoma	From decay of minerals containing uranium; potentially serious hazard in quarries and underground mines
Vinyl chloride	Hapatic angiosarcoma	Refrigerant; monomer for vinyl polymers; adhesive for plastics; formerly inert aerosol propellant in pressurized containers

Table 8.
Occupational cancers.

- DNA damage that is responsible for carcinogenicity.
- DNA damage is repaired by the nucleotide excision repair pathway.
- With excessive sun exposure, the DNA damage exceeds the capacity of the nucleotide excision repair pathway and genomic injury becomes mutagenic and carcinogenic.
- Xeroderma pigmentosum: It is a rare hereditary autosomal recessive disorder characterized by congenital deficiency of nucleotide excision repair DNA. These individuals develop skin cancers (basal cell carcinoma, squamous cell carcinoma, and melanoma) due to impairment in the excision of UV-damaged DNA [21, 22].

Ionizing radiation:

Electromagnetic (x-rays, γ-rays) and particulate (α particles, β particles, protons, neutrons) radiations are all carcinogenic.

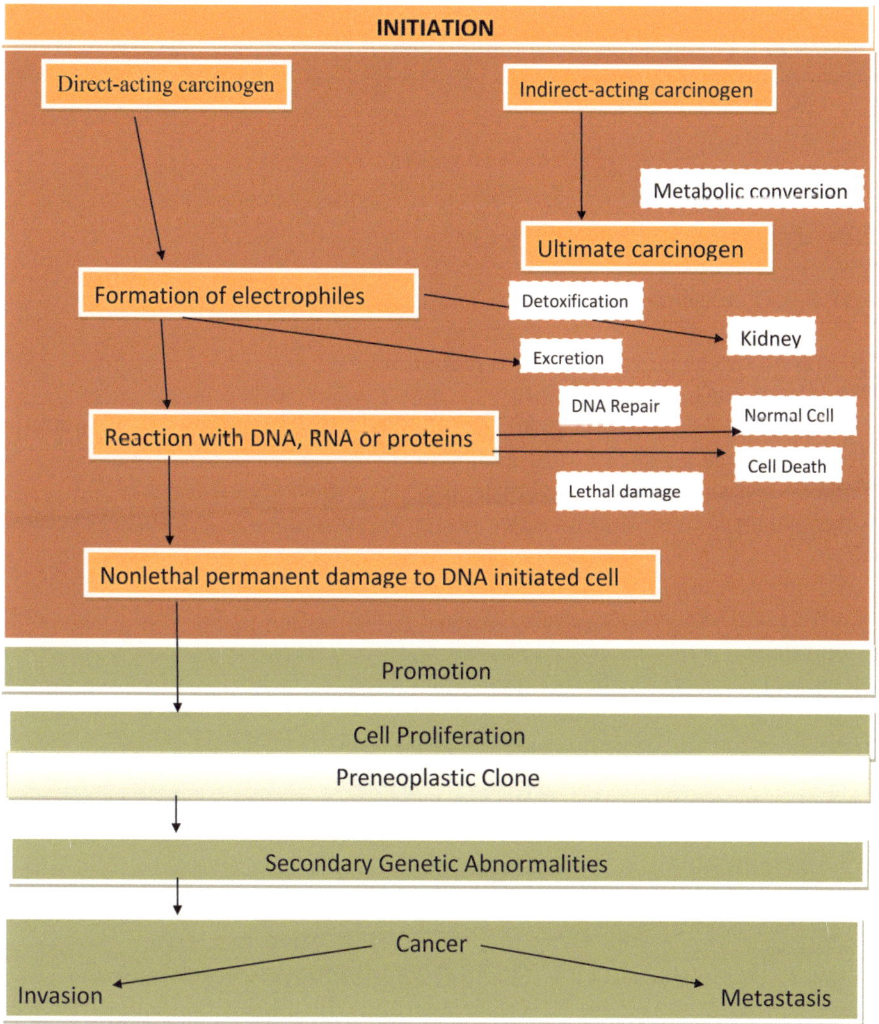

Figure 2.
Multistep theory of chemical carcinogenesis.

Cancers produced:
Medical or occupational exposure, for example., leukemia and skin cancers.
Nuclear plant accidents: Risk of lung cancers.
Atomic bomb explosion: Survivors of atomic bomb explosion (dropped on Hiroshima and Nagasaki) -› increased incidence of leukemia -> mainly acute and chronic myelogenous leukemia after about seven years.
Subsequently, increased mortality due to solid tumors (e.g., breast, colon, thyroid, and lung).

Therapeutic radiation:

1. Papillary carcinoma of the thyroid follows irradiation of head and neck and

2. Angiosarcoma of liver due to radioactive thorium dioxide used to visualize the arterial tree.

Mechanism: Hydroxyl free radical injury to DNA.

Tissues that are relatively resistant to radiation-induced neoplasia: Skin, bone, and the gastrointestinal tract.

UV rays cause skin cancer:

1. Squamous cell carcinoma.

2. Basal cell carcinoma.

3. Malignant melanoma.

Lymphoid tissue: most sensitive to radiation.

Bone: least sensitive to radiation.

UV radiation: induces formation of pyridine dimers in DNA leading to mutations.

Acute leukemia: most frequent malignant tumor caused by radiation.

Total body radiation: lymphopenia is the first hematological feature.

Xeroderma pigmentosum is caused due to abnormalities in nucleotide excision repair.

Ionizing radiation: Damages DNA.

Ionizing radiation causes genetic damage which cannot be repaired by nucleotide excision repair.

Neoplasm associated with therapeutic radiation.

1. Papillary carcinoma of thyroid.

2. Angiosarcoma of liver [21, 22].

8. Microbial carcinogenesis

Viruses that cause tumors are called as oncogenic viruses.

Many viruses have been proven to be oncogenic in animals, but only a few have been associated with human cancer.

Classification (Flowchart): They are mainly classified depending on the genetic material into:

1. Oncogenic RNA viruses, and

2. Oncogenic DNA viruses.

Mechanism: It is similar to that of HBV and HCV-induced hepatocellular carcinoma (**Table 9**).

Bacteria:-

Helicobacter pylori:

Diseases caused by *H. pylori* are (1) peptic ulcers, (2) gastric adenocarcinomas, and (3) gastric lymphomas, gastric adenocarcinomas.

- Chronic inflammation: *H. pylori* causes chronic inflammation (chronic gastritis) - > followed by gastric atrophy - > intestinal metaplasia -> dysplasia - > cancer,

- Genes: *H. pylori* causing gastric adenocarcinoma contains cytotoxin-associated A (CagA) gene that can penetrate into gastric epithelial cells - > initiation of signals - > unregulated growth factor stimulation.

Gastric lymphoma:

H. pylori produces lymphoma of B-cell origin, which are called as lymphomas of mucosa-associated lymphoid tissue or maltomas. *H. pylori* is associated with translocation in MALT lymphomas.

Fungi:

Fungi may cause cancer by producing toxic substances (mycotoxins). Aflatoxin B, produced by Aspergillus flavus is a potent carcinogen responsible for hepatocellular carcinoma.

Parasites:

Two parasites that can cause tumors are:

1. Schistosoma is strongly implicated in carcinoma of urinary bladder (usually of squamous cell type). The ova of the parasite can be found in the affected tissue.

2. *Clonorchis sinensis* (Chinese liver fluke) lodges in the bile ducts -> produces an inflammatory reaction, epithelial hyperplasia, and sometimes adenocarcinoma of the bile ducts (Cholangiocarcinoma).

Type of virus	**Lesions**
Oncogenic RNA	Viruses
• Human T-cell lymphotropic virus type-1	Adult T-cell leukemia/lymphoma
• Hepatitis C virus	Hepatocellular carcinoma
Oncogenic DNA	Viruses
1. Human papilloma virus	
A. Low-oncogenic risk HPV-benign	lesions of squamous epithelium
• HPV types 1, 2, 4 and 7	Benign squamous papilloma (wart)
• HPV-6 and HPV-11	Condylomata acuminata (genital warts) of the vulva, penis and perianal region
	Laryngeal papillomas
B. High-oncogenic risk HPV-	malignant tumors
• HPV types 16 and 18	Squamous cell carcinoma of the cervix and anogenital region
	Oropharyngeal cancers (tonsil)
2. Epstein-Barr virus	Burkitt lymphoma (requires cofactor-malaria)
	Nasopharyngeal cancer
3. Hepatitis B virus	Hepatocellular carcinoma
4. Human herpes virus-8	Kaposi's sarcoma
	Pleural effusion lymphoma, multicentric Castleman disease
5. Merkel cell polyomavirus	Merkel cell carcinoma

Table 9.
Various viruses implicated in human tumors and associated lesions.

Hormones:
Hormones in the body may act as cofactors in carcinogenesis.
Estrogen.

- Endometrial carcinoma: It may develop in females with estrogen-secreting granulosa cell tumor of ovary or those receiving exogenous estrogen.

- Adenocarcinoma of vagina: Increased frequency of adenocarcinoma of vagina is observed in daughters of mothers who received estrogen during pregnancy. Abnormal vascularity of tumor: Estrogens can make existing tumors abnormally vascular (e.g., adenomas and focal nodular hyperplasia).

- Androgenic and anabolic steroids: They may cause hepatocellular tumors.

- Hormone-dependent tumors.

- Prostatic carcinoma usually responds to administration of estrogens or castration.

- Breast carcinomas regress following oophorectomy.

- Microbial carcinogens: Viruses > bacteria > parasites [23–26].

9. Laboratory diagnosis of cancer

Confirmation of lesion as neoplastic usually requires cytological and/or histopathological examination of the suspected organ or tissue. Different laboratory methods available for the diagnosis of malignant tumors are:

9.1 Morphological methods

9.1.1 Histopathological examination

Histopathological diagnosis is based on the microscopic features of neoplasm and by this method of examination, accurate diagnosis can be made in majority of cases.

Clinical data: It should be provided for accurate pathologic diagnosis, for example:

- Radiation causes changes in the skin, which mimic changes seen in cancer.

- Sections taken from the site of a healing fracture can mimic an osteosarcoma.

- Adequate and representative area of the specimen should be sent.

Proper fixation [27–29].

9.1.2 Frozen section

In this method, tissue is hardened rapidly by freezing (hence termed frozen section) and sections are cut by special instrument called freezing microtome or cryostat (microtome in a refrigerated chamber). Its uses are:

- Rapid diagnosis: Frozen section is used for quick histologic diagnosis (within minutes) and is useful for determining the nature of a tumor (benign or malignant) lesion, especially when the patient is still on the operation table. It will help to determine whether a lesion is a neoplasm and, if so, whether it is benign or malignant.

- Evaluation of the margins of an excised cancer to know whether excision of the neoplasm is complete. If resection margins are inadequate, additional tissue can be removed immediately, without the need for a subsequent operation.

- Demonstration of fat mainly in nonneoplastic lesions.

- To know the lymph node (sentinel) status in carcinoma, knowing the extent of regional tumor metastases may be useful in deciding the further surgery.

- To determine whether additional workup is necessary for a particular tissue specimen while it is still fresh. For example, if the metastatic tumor found in a lymph node is recognized as a poorly differentiated carcinoma, special fixation and electron microscopy may be needed for proper diagnosis.

Various techniques for tissue sampling a Weddle biopsy: It is called a cutting-needle or core.

- Needle oriel biopsy. Using cutting needle, a core of this seems wide and 2 cm long is obtained for histologic examinations or special studies that permit evaluation of architectural structure. Tissue obtained is small and interpretation may be difficult.

- Endoscopy biopsy: It is performed through endoscopy. Usually performed for lesions in gastrointestinal, respiratory, urinary, and genital tracts.

- Incision biopsy: In this, the representative tissue sample is obtained by incising the lesions. Incisional biopsy (along with fine-needle aspiration) is often the method of choice for inoperable lesions, too large for excision, or when excision causes functional or cosmetic impairment.

- Excision biopsy: In this, entire abnormal lesion is surgically removed. It provides generous amounts of tissue for diagnosis and may be surgical therapy for some tumors (e.g., small- to medium-sized breast cancers).

Pitfalls in biopsy interpretation: These include inadequate tissue sampling and artifacts due to procedure itself (e.g. thermal damage caused by an electrocautery or laser) [27–29].

9.1.3 Cytological examination

It is performed on many tissues and is usually done for identifying neoplastic cells.

Methods of obtaining cells.

Exfoliative cytology: It is the study of spontaneously exfoliated (shed) cells from the lining of an organ into a body cavity.

Fine-needle aspiration cytology.

It involves aspiration of cells and attendant fluid with a small-bore needle. The smears are prepared and stained, followed by microscopic examination of cells. It is a widely-used simple and quick procedure.

Liquid-based cytology (thin prep): This is a special technique for preparation of samples that provides uniform monolayered dispersion of cells on smears.

Cytological characteristics of cancer cells:

Cancer cells have decreased cohesiveness and show cellular features of anaplasia. Cytological, differentiation can be made between normal, dysplastic, carcinoma in situ, and malignant cells.

Disadvantages of cytological examination:

Diagnosis is based on the features of individual cells or a clump of cells, without the supporting evidence of loss of orientation.

The invasion that is diagnostic of malignant tumor under histology cannot be assessed by cytology [27–29].

9.1.4 Histochemistry and cytochemistry

These are stains, which identify the chemical nature of cell contents or their products. H&E staining cannot demonstrate certain specific substances/constituents of cells. This requires some special stains. Common histochemical and cytochemical stains useful in diagnosis of tumors are listed in

Immunohistochemistry:-

It is an immunological method of identifying the antigenic component in the cell or one of its components by using specific antibodies. It is widely used in the diagnosis or management of malignant neoplasms.

Uses of Immunohistochemistry:-

To categorize undifferentiated cancers:

Many malignant tumors of diverse origins resemble each other and are difficult to distinguish on routine hematoxylin and eosin (H&E) sections.

Example: Few anaplastic carcinomas, lymphomas, melanomas, and sarcomas may look almost similar. They should be accurately diagnosed because of their different modes of treatment and prognosis.

- In poorly differentiated carcinoma, intermediate filaments (e.g., cytokeratins) show positivity.

- Malignant melanomas when unpigmented (amelanotic melanoma) appear similar to other poorly differentiated carcinomas. They express HMB-45 and S-100 protein, but negative for cytokeratins.

- Desmin is found in neoplasms of muscle cell origin.

- To determine the origin of poorly differentiated metastatic tumors: It may be determined by using tissue-specific or organ-specific antigens.

For prognosis or to select the mode of treatment:

- Identification of hormone (estrogen/progesterone) receptors in breast cancer cells is of prognostic and therapeutic value. These cancers respond well to antiestrogen therapy and have a better prognosis.

- Breast cancers with BRBB2 protein (HER2/neu) positivity have a poor prognosis [27–29].

9.1.5 Immunohistochemical markers

Apart from the various immunochemical markers mentioned above, other markers useful are as follows:

- Neuroendocrine tumors show positivity for cytokeratins like carcinomas, but they can be identified by their contents, namely:

- Chromogranins (proteins found in neurosecretory granules).

- Neuron-specific enolase (NSE).

- Synaptophysin.

- Soft tissue sarcomas: They show intermediate filament positivity.

- Vimenttin used to identify mesenchyme.

- Desmin is positive in smooth or striated muscle fibers.

- Muscle-specific actin marker for muscle tissue.

- Neurofilament proteins: Marker for tumors of neurons, neuroblastoma, and ganglioneuroma.

- Neuron-specific enolase in neuroblastoma.

- Glial fibrillary acidic protein (GFAP), also intermediate filament expressed in glial cell neoplasms.

- Malignant lymphomas: Generally positive for leukocyte common antigen (LCA, CD45). Markers for lymphomas and leukemias are called cluster designations (CDs) and are useful to differentiate T and B lymphocytes, monocytes, granulocytes and the mature and immature variants of these cells.

- Vascular tumors derived from endothelial cells include benign hemangiomas and malignant angiosarcomas, and are positive for factor VIII-related antigens or certain lectins.

- Proliferating cells: Cells in cell cycle show positivity for Ki-67 and proliferating cell nuclear antigen (PCNA) [27–29].

9.1.6 Electron microscopy

It helps in the diagnosis of poorly differentiated/undifferentiated cancers, which cannot identify the origin by light microscopy, for example, carcinomas show desmosomes and specialized junctional complexes, structures that are not seen in sarcomas or lymphomas [27–29].

9.1.7 Flow cytometry

It quantitatively measures various individual cell characteristics, such as membrane antigens and the DNA content of tumor cells. Flow cytometry is useful for identification and classification of tumors of T and B lymphocytes (leukemias and lymphomas) and mononuclear-phagocytic cells.

Circulating tumor cells.

Detection, quantification, and characterization of rare solid tumor cells (e.g., carcinoma and melanoma) circulating in the blood are emerging as a diagnostic modality, although presently in the research stage. Few latest devices detect three-dimensional flow cells coated with antibodies specific for tumor cells of interest (e.g., carcinoma cells) in the blood.

It will be useful for early diagnosis, assessing the risk of metastasis, and assessing the response of tumor cells to therapy.

Tumor makers:

Tumor markers are products of malignant tumors that can be detected in the cells themselves or in blood and body fluids.

Usefulness

- Detection of cancer, for example, PSA is the most common and useful tumor marker used to screen prostatic adenocarcinoma. High levels of PSA are found in the blood of prostatic carcinoma patients but it also may be elevated in benign prostatic hyperplasia.
- Determine the effectiveness of therapy.
- Detection of recurrence.

9.2 Molecular profiling of tumors

9.2.1 Traditional cancer typing

Traditionally cancer is diagnosed and classified according to the morphological (histopathology/ cytopathology) appearance of the cells and their surrounding tissue. It has limitations such as (i) relies on a subjective review of the tissue, which is dependent on the knowledge and experience of a pathologist, and, therefore, may not be reproducible, (ii) limited ability to determine the individual recurrence risk of cancer, (iii) insufficient to reflect the complicated underlying molecular events that drive the neoplastic process, and (iv) histopathology reports lack or offer very little information regarding the potential drug treatment regime to which cancer will respond. Traditional pathology reports help to determine treatment that leads to better outcomes. However, tumors with identical pathology may have different origins and respond differently to a treatment.

Newer cancer diagnostics:-

1. DNA microarray

2. DNA sequencing [27–29]

10. Tumor markers

Tumor markers are products of malignant tumors tar fun be detected in the cells themselves or in blood and body fluids.

Usefulness:

1. Detection of cancer, for example PSA is the most common and useful tumor marker used to screen prostatic adenocarcinoma. High levels of PA are found in the blood of prostatic carcinoma patients but it also may be elevated in benign prostatic hyperplasia.

2. Determine the effectiveness of therapy.

3. Detection of recurrence.

Types of markers (Table): These may be tumor-associated hormones, oncofetal antigens, specific proteins, mucin and glycoproteins, enzymes, and molecular markers.

Molecular diagnosis:

Molecular diagnosis can be done by different techniques such as FISH technique and PCR (polymerase chain reaction) analysis.

10.1 Diagnosis of cancer

- Monoclonal (malignant) versus polyclonal (benign): To differentiate benign (polyclonal) proliferations of T-or B-cells from malignant (monoclonal) proliferations.

- Chromosomal alterations: Many hematopoietic neoplasms (leukemias and lymphomas) and few solid tumors (e.g. Ewings Sarcoma) are characterized by particular translocations that can be detected by FISH technique or by PCR analysis [27–29].

10.2 Prognosis of cancer

Certain genetic alterations are of prognostic value. They can be detected by routine cytogenetics and also by FISH or PCR assays. Example of poor prognostic feature is amplification of tie N-MIC gene and deletions of IP in neuroblastoma and amplification of HER-2/Neu in breast cancer.

10.3 Detection of minimal residual disease

Prognosis of cancer can detect minimal residual disease or the onset of relapse in patients who are treated for leukemia or lymphoma, for example, detection of BCR-ABL transcripts in treated patients with CML.

10.4 Detection of hereditary predisposition to cancer

Germline mutations in many tumor suppressor genes are associated with increased risk for specific cancers. This will help in prophylactic surgery and counseling of relatives at risk, for example, BRCAI, BRCA2, and the RET protooncogene.

For therapeutic decision, It is useful in target therapy [27–29] (**Table 10**).

10.5 Molecular profiling of tumors

10.5.1 Traditional cancer typing

Traditionally cancer is diagnosed and classified according to the morphological (histopathology/cytopathology) appearance of the cells and their surrounding tissue. It has limitations such as (1) it relies on a subjective review of the tissue, which is dependent on the knowledge and experience of a pathologist, and, therefore, may not be reproducible, (2) Limited ability to determine the individual recurrence risk of cancer, (3) Insufficient to reflect the complicated underlying molecular events that drive the neoplastic process and (4) Histopathology reports lack or offer very little information regarding the potential drug treatment regime to which cancer will respond. Traditional pathology reports help to determine treatment that leads to better outcomes. However, tumors with identical pathology may have different origins and respond differently to treatment.

10.5.2 Clinical aspects of neoplasia

Both benign and malignant tumors may produce clinical features through their various effects on host.

Local effects:-.

These are due to encroachment on adjacent structures.

- Compression (e.g. adenoma in the ampulla of Vater causing obstruction of biliary tract).

- Mechanical obstruction: It may be caused by both benign and malignant tumors. Example: Tumors may cause obstruction or intussusception in the GI tract.

- “Endocrine insufficiency: It is caused due to destruction of an endocrine gland either due to primary or metastatic cancer.

- Ulceration, bleeding, and secondary infections: It may develop in benign or malignant tumors in the skin or mucosa of the GI tract, for example.

- Melena (blood in the stool) in neoplasms of the gut.

- Hematuria in neoplasms of the urinary tract.

“Rupture” or infarction of tumor.

Functional effects:-.

These include:

- Hormonal effects: It may be observed both in benign and malignant tumors of endocrine glands, for example, B-cell adenoma of the pancreas may produce insulin -› to cause fatal hypoglycemia.

Clnical sydromes	Major forms of underlying cancer	Causal mechanism
Endocrinopathies		
Cushing syndrome	Small-cell carcinoma of lung pancreatic carcinoma neural tumors	ACTH or ACTH-like substance
Syndrome of inappropriate antidiuretic hormone secretion	Small-cell carcinoma of lung intracranial neoplasms	Antidiuretic hormone or atrial natriuretic hormones
Hypercalcemia	Squamous cell carcinoma of lung breast carcinoma renal carcinoma adult T-cell leukemia/lymphoma	Parathyroid hormoine-related protein (PTHRP), TGF-a, TNF, IL-1
Hypoglycemia	Ovarian carcionama fibrosarcoma other mesenchymal sarcomas	Insulin or insufin-like substance
Polycythemia	Renal carcinoma cerebellar hemangioma hapatocellular carcinoma	Eryhropoietin
Nerve and muscle syndromes		
Myasthenia	Bronchogenic carcinoma thymic neoplasms	Immunologic
Disorders of the central and peripheral nervous system	Breast carcinoma	
Dermatologic disorders		
Acanthosis nignicans	Gastric carcinoma lung carcinoma utierine carcinoma	Immunologic; secretion of epidermal growth factor
Dermatomyositis	Bronchogenic carcinoma breast carcinoma	Immunologic
Osseous, articular, and soft tissue changes		
Hypertophic osteoarthropathy and clubbing of the fingers	Bronchogenic carcinoma Thymic neoplasms	Unknown
Vascular and hematologic changes		
Venous thrombosis (Trousseau phenomenon)	Pancreatic carcinoma bronchogenic carcinoma Other cancers	Tumor products (mucins that acticate clotting)
Disseminated thrombotic endocarditis	Acute promyelocytic leukemia prostatic carcinoma	Tumor products that acticate clotting
Nonbacterial thrombotic endocarditis	Advanced cancers	Hypercoagulability
Red call aplasia	Thymic neoplasms	Unknown
Others		
Nephrotic syndrome	Various cancers	Tumor antigens, immune complexes

Table 10.
Paraneoplastic syndiomes.

- Paraneoplastic syndromes: Non endocrine tumors may secrete hormones or hormone-like substances and produce paraneoplastic syndromes (explained below).
- Fever: It is most commonly associated with Hodgkin disease, renal cell carcinoma, and osteogenic sarcoma. Fever may be due to release of pyogenes by tumor cells or IL-1 produced by inflammatory cells in the stroma of the tumor [30–32].

10.5.3 Tumor lysis syndrome

- It is a group of metabolic complications that can occur after treatment for leukemias such as acute lymphoblastic leukemia (ALL) and chronic lymphocytic leukemias (CLL), lymphomas such as Burkitt lymphoma, and uncommonly in solid tumors.
- It is caused by breakdown products of tumor cells following chemotherapy or glucocorticoids or hormonal agent (tamoxifen).
- The killed tumor cells release intracellular ions and large amounts of metabolic byproducts into systemic circulation.
- Metabolic abnormalities include:
- Hyperuricemia: Due to increased turnover of nucleic acids. It can cause uric acid precipitation in the kidney resulting in renal failure.
- Hyperkalemia: Due to release of the most abundant intracellular cation potassium.
- Hyperphosphatemia: Due to release of intracellular phosphate.
- Hypocalcemia: Due to complexing of calcium with elevated phosphate.
- Lactic acidosis [30–32].
- Cancer cachexia (wasting):-
- It is defined as progressive weight loss accompanied by severe weakness, anorexia, and anemia developing in patients with cancer.
- Mechanism: It is poorly understood and may be due to TNF and other cytokines, like IL-1, interferon-y, and leukemia inhibitory factor. They may be produced by macrophages in the tumor or by the tumor cells themselves [30–32].

11. Tumor staging and granding

11.1 TNM staging systems

It is the cancer staging system that is widely used and varies for each specific form of cancer. Its general principles are:

- T refers to the size of the primary tumor.
- It is suffixed by a number that indicates the size of the tumor or local anatomical extent. The number varies according to the organ involved in the tumor. With increasing size, the primary lesion is characterized as TI to T4.
- T0 is used to denote an in situ lesion.
- Refers to lymph node status.

- It is suffixed by a number to indicate the number of regional lymph nodes or groups of lymph nodes showing metastases.
- N0 would mean no nodal involvement.
- M refers to the presence and anatomical extent of distant metastases.
- M0 signifies no distant metastases, whereas
- M1 indicates the presence of metastases.

TNM staging system is widely used.
TNM staging.

- T = size of primary tumor.
- N = lymph node status.
- M = metastatic status [30–32].

Grading of tumor depends on the degree of differentiation.

Prognosis of tumor depends on:

1. Histological type.
2. Grade.
3. Stage.

11.2 Prognosis

The prognosis of malignant tumors varies and is determined partly by the characteristics of the tumor cells (e.g. grower pale invasiveness) and partly by the effectiveness of therapy [30–32].

12. Paraneoplastic syndromes

Malignant tumors invade local tissue, produce metastasis, and can produce a variety of products that can stimulate hormonal, hematologic, dermatologic, and neurologic responses.

Definition: Paraneoplastic syndromes are symptom complexes in cancer patients that are not directly related to mass effects or invasion or metastasis or by the secretion of hormones indigenous to the tissue of origin.

Frequency: Though they occur in 10–15% of patients, it is important because:

1. Maybe the first manifestation of an occult neoplasm.
2. Maybe mistaken for metastatic disease leading to inappropriate treatment.
3. May present clinical problems, which may be fatal.

Tumor markers	Tumor types
Harmones	
Human chorionic gonadotropin	Trophoblastic tumors, nonseminomatous testicular tumors
Calcitonin	Medullary carcinoma of thyroid
Catecholamine and metabolites	Pheochromocytoma and related tumors
Ectopic hormones	See table 7-11
Oncofetal antigens	
a-Fetoprotein	Liver cell cancer, nonseminomatous germ cell tumors of testis
Carcinoembryonic antigen	Carcinomas of the colon, pancreas, lung, stomach, and heart
Isoenzymes	
Prostatic acid phosphatase	Prostate cancer
Neuron-specific enolase	Small-cell cancer of lung, neuroblastoma
Specific proteins	
Immunoglobulins	Multiple myeloma and other gammopathies
Prostate-specific antigen and prostate-specific membrane antigen	Prostate cancer
Mucins and other glycoproteins	
CA-125	Ovarian cancer
CA-19-9	Colon cancer, pancreatic cancer
CA-15-3	Breast cancer
Cell-free DNA markers	
TP53, APC RAS mutants in stool and sarum	Colon cancer
TP53, RAS mutants in stool and serum	pancreatic cancer
TP53, RAS mutants in sputum and sermu	Lung cancer
TP53 mutants in urine	Bladder cancer

Table 11.
Selected tumor markers.

4. Certain tumor products causing paraneoplastic syndromes may be useful in monitoring recurrence in patients who had surgical resections or are undergoing chemotherapy or radiation therapy.

Some paraneoplastic syndromes, their mechanism, and the common cancers causing them are listed in **Table 11** [30–32].

13. Conclusion

With all the advances in genomic analyzes and targeted therapies, it can be safely predicted that we are on the cusp of a golden age of tumor diagnosis and treatment.

DOI: http://dx.doi.org/10.5772/intechopen.109512

Those of you now in medical school can safely assume that expectations of rapid advances in cancer diagnosis and therapy will be fulfilled while you are still in practice.

Author details

Flora Thanadar Ajmiree
Dr. Sirajul Islam Medical College and Hospital, Dhaka, Bangladesh

*Address all correspondence to: ajmiree.flora2020@gmail.com

References

[1] Kumar V, Abbas AK, Aster JC. Robbins Basic Pathology. 10th ed. Jeremy Bowes, ELSEVIER, (A Division of Reed Elsevier India Pvt. Ltd.); 2021

[2] de Martel C, Ferlay J, Franceschi S, et al. Global burden of cancers attributable to infections in 2008: A review and synthetic analysis. The Lancet Oncology. 2012;**13**:607-615. [A recent analysis that estimates that approximately 16% of cancers (2 million cases per year) are attributable to infectious agents]

[3] Faulds MH, Dahlman-Wright K. Metabolic diseases and cancer risk. Current Opinion in Oncology. 2012;**24**: 58-61. [A review focused on evidence linking metabolic disorders such obesity and diabetes to increased cancer risk]

[4] Liang J, Shang Y. Estrogen and cancer. Annual Review of Physiology. 2013;**75**:225-240. [A summary of epidemiologic evidence connecting hyperestrogen-ism to cancer and of current understanding of the oncogenic mechanisms of estrogen signaling]

[5] Roberts DL, Dive C, Renehan AG. Biological mechanisms linking obesity and cancer risk: New perspectives. Annual Re Medicine. 2010;**61**:301-316 [Discussion of possible biological processes that increase cancer risk in the obese]

[6] Hanahan D, Weinberg RA. Hallmarks of cancer: The next generation. Cell. 2011;**144**:646-674. [An update of a classic paper describing the key features common to all cancers]

[7] Cilloni D, Saglio G. Molecular pathways: BCR-ABL. Clinical Cancer Research. 2012;**18**:930-937. [A discussion of the functional consequences and clinical significance of aberrant tyrosine kinase activity in chronic myeloid leukemia mediated by the constitutive enzyme activity of BCR-ABL]

[8] Dang CV. MYC on the path to cancer. Cell. 2012;**149**:22-35. [A review of the widespread oncogenic role. of the transcription factor MYC in cancer!]

[9] Pao W, Chmielecki J. Rational, biologically based treatment of EGFR-mutant non-small-cell lung cancer. Natural Red Cancer. 2010;**10**:760-774. [A review summarizing recent work aimed at treating and ultimately curing lung cancers associated with activating mutations in the receptor tyrosine kinase EGFR]

[10] Pylayeva-Gupta Y, Grabocka E, Bar-Sagi D. RAS oncogenes: Weaving a tumorigenic web. Natural Review Cancer. 2011;**11**:761-774. [A description of how RAS oncogenes activate multiple downstrean signaling pathonys to drive cellular transformation and oncogenesis]

[11] Goh AM, Coffill CR, Lane DP. The role of mutant p53 in human cancer. Pathology. 2011;**223**:116-126. [Discussion of emerging oncogenic roles of mutant p53 proteins]

[12] Manning AL, Dyson NJ. RB: Mitotic implications of a tumour suppres sor. Natural Review Cancer. 2012;**12**:220-226. [In addition to the well established roles of RB in control of cell cycle progression and proliferation, this review describes other emerging tumor suppressive functions, such as maintenance of genomic stability]

[13] Roy R, Chun J, Powell SN. BRCA1 and BRCA2: Different roles in a common pathway of genome protection. Natural

Review Cancer. 2012;**12**:68-78. [A discussion of the concerted roles of the BRCA1 and BRCA2 tumor suppressor proteins in protecting the genore from double-strand DNA damage during DNA replication]

[14] Song MS, Salmena L, Pandolfi PP. The functions and regulation of the PTEN tumour suppressor. Natural Review in Molecular Cell Biology. 2012; **13**:283-296. [A detailed discussion of the tumor suppressive role of the the lipid phos phatase PTEN]

[15] Ward PS, Thompson CB. Metabolic reprogramming: A cancer halt mark even warburg did not anticipate. Cancer Cell. 2012;**21**:297-308. [A review making the case that altered cancer metabolism is a fundamental hallmark of cancer cells]

[16] Spano D, Heck C, De Antonellis P, et al. Molecular networks that regulate cancer metastasis. Seminars in Cancer Biology. 2012;**22**:234-249. [A review that addresses some of the genetic events and critical factors that contributes to acquisition of the metastatic phenotype during oncogenesis]

[17] Tiwari N, Gheldof A, Tatari M, et al. EMT as the ultimate survival mechanism of cancer cells. Seminars in Cancer Biology. 2012;**22**:194-207. [A far-ranging discussion of the possible roles of epithelinl-mesenchymal transition in metastasis and other cancer hallmarks]

[18] Lozy F, Karantza V. Autophagy and cancer cell metabolism. Seminars in Cancer Biology. 2012;**23**:395-401. [A discussion of how cellular metabolism and autophagy may contribute to the ability of cancer cells to adapt to environmental stressors and survive radiation and chemotherapy

[19] Mah LY, Ryan KM. Autophagy and cancer. Cold Springer Harbor Perspective Biology. 2012;**4**:a008821. [LA review of the possible interplay between autoph agy and various aspects of tumor suppression, including cellular responses to nutrient and hypoxic stress, control of programmed cell death, and tumor-associated immune responses]

[20] Brahmer JR, Tykodi SS, Chow LQ, et al. Safety and activity of anti-PD-Li antibody in patients with advanced cancer. New England Journal of Medicine. 2012; **366**:2455-2465. [Two back-to-back landmark papers describing the anti-cancer activity of antibodies that interfere with the activity of PD-1, a signaling receptor that inhibits T cell function]

[21] Berger MF, Hodis E, Heffernan TP, et al. Melanoma genome sequene ing reveals frequent PREX2 mutations. Nature. 2012;**485**:502-506. [A study that describes and quantifies the mutational impact of sun-exposure on melanoma genomes]

[22] Pleasance ED, Stephens PJ, O'Meara S, et al. A small-cell lung cancer genome with complex signatures of tobacco exposure. Nature. 2010;**463**: 184-190. [A study that describes and quantifies the mutational impact of carcinogens in tobacco smoke on lung cancer genomes]

[23] Cabibbo G, Maida M, Genco C, et al. Causes of and prevention strate gies for hepatocellular carcinoma. Seminars in Oncology. 2012;**39**:374-383. [A discussion of the various environmental factors implicated in hepato cellular carcinoma, including hepatitis viruses]

[24] Magrath I. Epidemiology: Clues to the pathogenesis of Burkitt lyn phoma. British Journal of Haematology. 2012; **156**:744-756. [A discussion of the roles of Epstein-Barr virus and malaria in genesis of this agressive B cell malignancy]

[25] Moody CA, Laimins LA. Human papillomavirus oncoproteins: Path - ways to transformation. Nat Re. Cancer. 2010;**10**:550-560. [A review focused on the oncogenic activities of HPV E6 and E7 proteins]

[26] Peleteiro B, La Vecchia C, Lunet N. The role of helicobacter pylori infection in the web of gastric cancer causation. Cancer Prevention. 2012;**21**:118-125. [A review that proposes a conceptual framework for understanding the role of *H. pylori* infection in gastric cancer]

[27] Alix-Panabieres C, Schwarzenbach H, Lantel K. Circulating tumor cells and circulating tumor DNA. Annual Review Medicine. 2012;**63**: 199-215. [A review discussing the detection, characterization, and diagnostic implications of rare circulating tumor cells and free nucleic acids derived from tumors]

[28] Kohlmann A, Grossmann V, Haferlach T. Integration of next-generation sequencing into clinical practice: Are we there yet? Seminars in Oncology. 2012;**39**:26-36. [A discussion of how and when deep sequencing may impact cancer diagnosis, therapy selection, and monitoring of response to therapy]

[29] Pao W, Lafrate AJ, Su Z. Genetically informed lung cancer medicine. Pathology. 2011;**223**:230-240. [A review of the rapid adoption and application of genomic analysis to the diagnosis and treatment of lung cancer]

[30] Azar L, Khasnis A. Paraneoplastic rheumatologic syndromes. Current Opinion in Rheumatology. 2013;**25**: 44-49. [A review focused on paraneoplastic sunovitis, bone disease, myositis, and vasculitis]

[31] Graus F, Dalmau I. Paraneoplastic neurological syndromes. Current Opinion in Neurology. 2012;**25**:795-801. [A review describing parancoplastic neurological syndromes and the impact of antibodies against surface antigens in their management]

[32] Lucia S, Esposito M, Rossi Fanelli F, et al. Cancer cachexia: From molecular mechanisms to patient's care. Critical Review Oncogology. 2012;**17**:315-321. [A review of cancer cachexia mechanisms and their implications for development of effective therapies]

Chapter 8

Perspective Chapter: Molecular Pathology of Lung Cancer

Shivani Gandhi, Ishani Gupta, Reetika Menia and Raman Kumar

Abstract

Lung cancers, due to delays in diagnosis and availability of limited treatment resources, have become the leading cause of cancer-related death globally. With the recent advances in the identification of molecular mechanisms and profile of lung cancer, the understanding of novel characteristics of the molecular pathology of lung cancers as well as knowledge of driver mutations has been enhanced that has led to the development and success of targeted strategies against lung cancer. Diagnosis and treatment of this heterogeneous group of cancer have been revolutionized with the advent of the identification of genetic alterations. This chapter will summarize the etiopathogenesis, current knowledge depicting the series of events associated with the development of lung cancer, the molecular mechanism of most common and relevant genetic alterations in lung cancer along with a brief about the use of targeted therapies in lung cancer patients.

Keywords: molecular, pathology, lung cancers, molecular mechanism, tumor suppressor genes

1. Introduction

Lung cancer is one of the most frequently diagnosed cancers worldwide and is the leading cause of cancer-related mortality, late diagnoses being one of the commonest reasons for this. A total of 13% of new cases of cancer as well as 19% of deaths related to cancer are attributed to lung cancers globally. A total of 1.8 million new cases of lung cancer were estimated in the year 2012. Cancer-related mortality due to lung cancer is common in men, with the highest number of cases being reported from Mizoram in both males and females (age-adjusted rate 28.3 and 28.7 per 100,000 population in males and females, respectively). A total of 6.9% of all new cases of cancer and 9.3% of deaths related to cancer are constituted by lung cancer alone in India in both men and women. The 5-year survival rate is less than 15%, despite significant advances in both diagnostic and therapeutic approaches [1–3].

With the identification of the molecular profile of lung cancer, the understanding of molecular pathology has also been enhanced. Many genetic alterations in the cancer stem cells have been revealed with the help of molecular studies and these cancer stem cells play an important role to produce clones of cancer cells to form tumor mass. Many genetic driver mutations have been identified with the help of combined genomic and transcriptomic sequencing studies and these driver mutations undergo stepwise accumulation resulting in the development of lung cancer. Molecular-targeted therapies have been identified to predict the response in patients of lung cancers to these targeted therapies with the advent and identification of driver mutations. The identification and knowledge of the molecular pathology of lung cancers have further led to the modification in the histological classification of cancers of the lung. A huge success rate has been observed in the development as well as approval of the targeted therapies and approach with the improved understanding in the identification of the genetic signature and the pathogenesis of molecular mechanism in approximately 20% of squamous cell carcinoma (SCC) and 60% of adenocarcinoma of lung. Dramatic response rates along with improved progression-free survival (PFS) have been observed with the use of targeted therapies in patients of lung cancers harboring mutations of genes like epidermal growth factor receptor (EGFR) or anaplastic lymphoma kinase (ALK) gene. Therefore, molecular testing is now being routinely used to guide the clinical care of lung cancer patients to predict one's therapeutic response [4–9].

Lung cancers have been classified into several histological subtypes based on the molecular profiles and targetable genetic alterations in lung cancer. It is a heterogeneous disease that shows variation in clinical features and biological behavior. Heterogeneity in the molecular mechanism reflects the molecular changes that occur in different subtypes of lung cancer. Genetic abnormalities associated with the development of cancer include a gain of function mutation of oncogenes like EGFR, BRAF, KRAS, AKL, MET, HER-2, loss of function mutation of tumor suppressor genes like TP53, PTEN, STK11, expression of growth factor, and their receptors. Targeted therapies are highly dependent upon molecular pathology; thus, the thorough understanding and knowledge of the molecular mechanism of different types of lung cancer is an integral part to understand the biological behavior and predict the response of cancer to the targeted therapy. With the identification of genetic mutations involved in particular cancer, the biological behavior of lung cancer can be determined which is essential for the diagnostic and therapeutic strategies that can target molecular aberrations.

In addition to the well-known genetic alterations in lung cancer that have been previously identified such as BRAF, EGFR & KRAS, many other genetic alterations such as ERBB2, RET, JAK2, DDR2 that occur in low frequency but are recurrent have also been identified with the help of genomic studies that have led to the development of targeted approach against lung cancers [10–13].

2. Etiology of lung cancer

In addition to cigarette smoking, which is one of the well-known carcinogens, there are many other environmental as well as genetic factors that contribute to lung cancer, discussed as under:

2.1 Smoking

Smoking alone accounts for approximately 90% cases of lung cancer and the risk is directly proportional to the duration of smoking and the number of cigarettes smoked/day. The risk of lung cancer is the same with cigar and pipe smoking as it is with cigarette smoking. Smoking of low-tar or "light" cigarettes also increases the risk of lung cancer as much as regular cigarettes. Menthol cigarette smoking increases the risk even more as menthol may allow people to inhale more deeply.

2.2 Secondhand smoke

With the passive smoking risk of lung cancer increases by 20 to 30%. More than 7000 deaths from lung cancer each year occur due to secondhand smoke.

2.3 Exposure to radon

Radon is a naturally occurring radioactive gas that is formed by the breakdown of uranium in soil and rocks. Uranium miners have small but significant risk of lung cancer due to exposure to radon. In Europe, 2% of all deaths from lung cancer in smokers were due to appreciable hazards from residential radon.

2.4 Exposure to asbestos

With exposure to asbestos, the risk of lung cancer is further increased and is seen more in smokers. The risk of lung cancer with asbestos exposure is directly proportional to the dose concentration and the type of asbestos fiber.

2.5 Exposure to other cancer-causing agents in the workplace

Metal exposure such as chromium, nickel, arsenic, and polycyclic aromatic hydrocarbons is also associated with lung cancer.

2.6 Previous radiation therapy to the lungs

Radiation exposure for non-lung cancer treatment, like non-Hodgkin's lymphoma and breast cancer, also increases the risk of lung cancer. Certain disorders of the lung like idiopathic pulmonary fibrosis increase the risk of lung cancer independent of smoking.

2.7 Air pollution

Air pollution is also an important risk factor for lung cancer. Around 5% of all deaths from lung cancer may occur due to outdoor air pollution worldwide.

2.8 Personal or family history of lung cancer

First-degree relatives of lung cancer patients have an increased risk to develop cancer.

2.9 Other lung diseases and airways obstruction

Some non-malignant diseases like COPD are associated with an increased risk for lung cancer. Tobacco smoking is the primary risk factor causing both lung cancer and COPD. Patients with interstitial fibrosis are at an increased risk of lung cancer.

2.10 Genetic factors

Susceptibility to lung cancer is determined by host genetic factors. Tobacco smokers with genetic susceptibility are at a higher risk.

3. Molecular mechanism of lung cancer

Molecular aberrations in oncogenes, proto-oncogenes as well as tumor suppressor genes have been recognized broadly in the pathogenesis of lung cancer. Gain of function mutation of oncogenes, and loss of function mutation of tumor suppressor genes result in the accumulation of multiple genetic abnormalities over a period of time that act by causing cellular alterations such as loss of function mutation of TP53, Rb genes is common in small-cell carcinoma whereas gain of function mutation of genes encoding tyrosine kinase receptors is seen in adenocarcinoma as depicted in **Figure 1**. Accumulation of multiple genetic abnormalities forms an initiating step for tumor progression. Some of the genetic alterations involved in lung cancer progression are discussed as follows.

4. Oncogene/proto oncogene

4.1 KRAS

KRAS is a member of the RAS family of proto-oncogenes, which also includes HRAS and NRAS. These three RAS genes encode monomeric GTPases that play a critical role in controlling the signal transduction pathways, regulate cell proliferation, differentiation, and cell survival. RAS proteins are bound to guanosine diphosphate (GDP) and are inactive in normal quiescent cells. On binding of the growth factor to the growth factor receptor, there is a transition to the active guanosine triphosphate (GTP) bound form that leads to the formation of an activated RAS-GTP complex, and this complex further bind to activate a number of other downstream signaling pathways such as RAF/MEK/MAPK/RAS PI3K/AKT pathways. Downstream signaling of pathways is initiated *via* KRAS incited by various growth factor receptors including EGFR and thus constitutive activation of this protein overcomes the need for growth

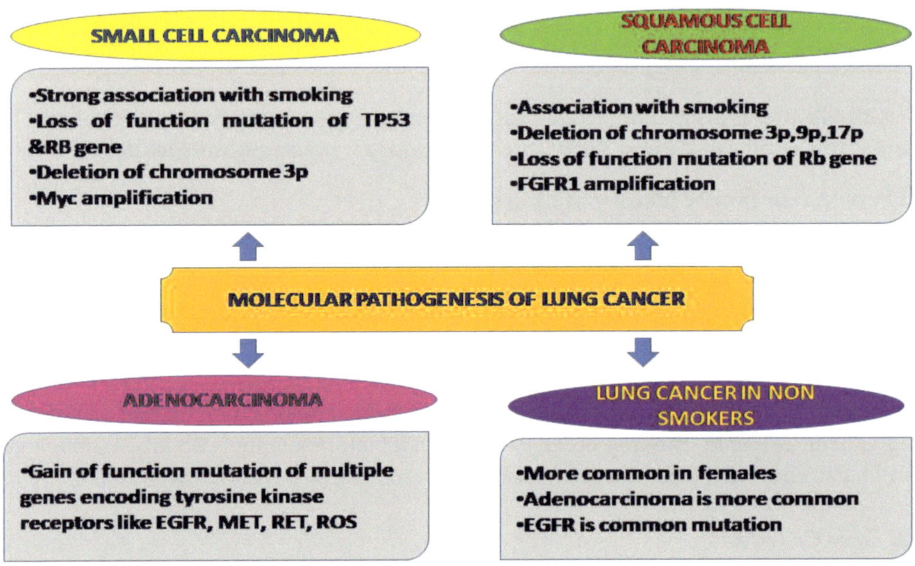

Figure 1.
Molecular pathogenesis of lung cancer.

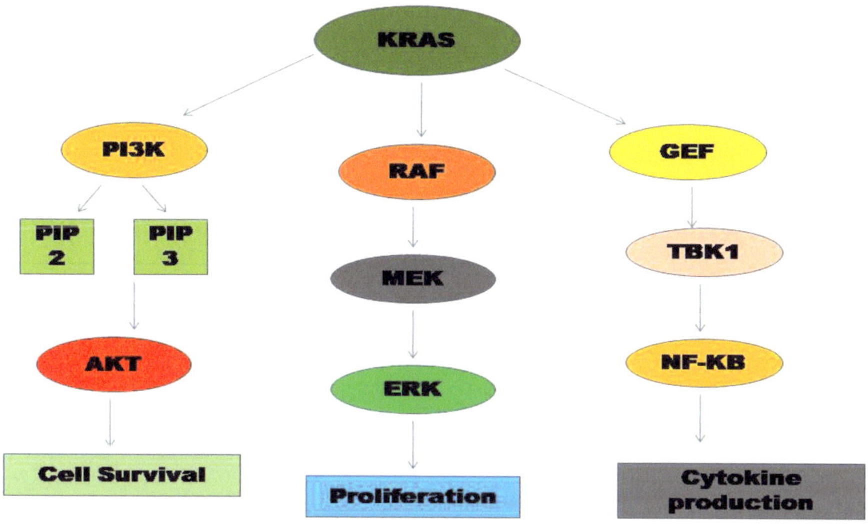

Figure 2.
KRAS effector pathway.

factor-mediated signaling. Activating RAS mutations alter the GTPase activity of the protein, thus hampering the inactivation of active RAS-GTP to GDP which leads to an increase in the downstream growth-promoting signaling pathway. In lung cancer, RAS/RAF/MEK/MAPK signal transduction cascade plays a pivotal role (**Figure 2**).

Activating KRAS mutation is the commonest oncogenic alteration in lung adenocarcinoma, which occurs in about 25–40% of cases, while mutations of HRAS and NRAS are very rare. KRAS mutation is more frequently observed in males and smokers. A total of 0–15% cases of adenocarcinoma in never smokers reported KRAS mutation. In squamous cell carcinoma or small-cell carcinoma, KRAS mutation is very rare or absent. KRAS mutations primarily occur at codon 12, occasionally at codon 13, and very rare at codon 61. The most common mutations in KRAS are G to T transversions (~84%) in smokers, while never smokers have G to A transitions.

EGFR and KRAS mutations are mutually exclusive, although there may be rare exceptions to this. A literature review has suggested that KRAS mutant tumors are resistant to the EGFR tyrosine kinase inhibitors (TKIs), as the mutations in KRAS lead to constitutive activation of the pathways, which are downstream of EGFR. In lung cancer, the high frequency of KRAS mutations makes it an ideal target for the treatment of cancer [14–23].

4.2 EGFR

EGFR is a member of erbB family having closely related receptor tyrosine kinases, which also includes erbB1 (also known as EGFR), erbB2 (HER2), erbB3, and erbB4. EGFR has an extracellular ligand binding domain, a transmembrane portion, and intracellular tyrosine kinase and regulatory domains. On binding of a specific ligand (e.g., epidermal growth factor), there occurs a conformational change and phosphorylation of the intracellular domain occurs, which leads to downstream signal transduction by various pathways that include PI3K/AKT/mTOR, RAS/RAF//MAPK, and JAK/STAT signaling pathways. Depending on the pathway undertaken, the end result is cell proliferation or cell maintenance by inhibition of apoptosis (**Figure 3**).

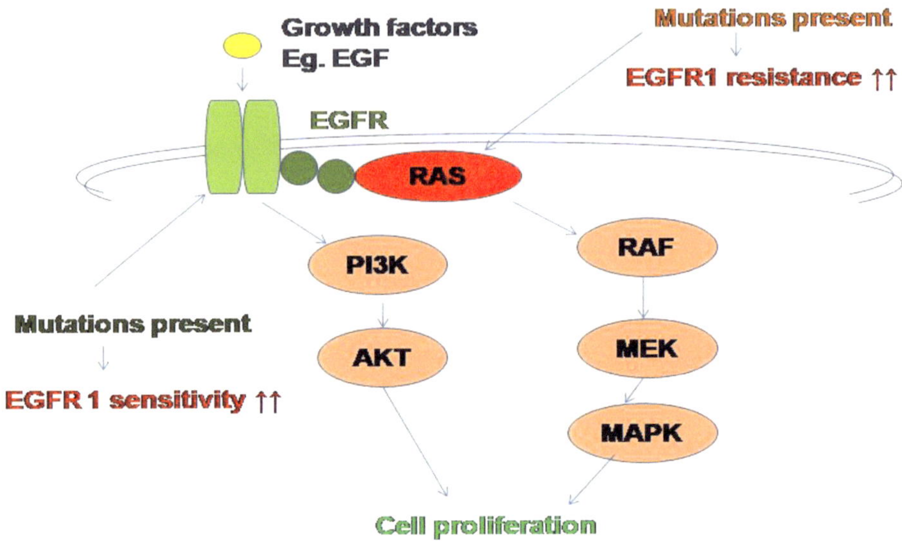

Figure 3.
EGFR signal transduction in cancer cells.

DNA mutations in EGFR can occur in the extracellular region or intracellular portions of the protein. In 43–89% cases of non-small-cell lung cancer, overexpression of EGFR or mutations in intracellular EGFR have been observed. Mutations in the EGFR tyrosine kinase domain are observed in around one-quarter of NSCLC and are associated with increased receptor expression in 75% of cases. Exon 19 frame deletions and exon 21 point mutation are the most common domain mutations in EGFR tyrosine kinase leading to the substitution of leucine at codon 858 in place of arginine, as a result of which signal transduction pathways get activated resulting in increased proliferation of cells and inhibition of apoptosis irrespective of the presence of ligand at extracellular site. Mutations in exons 18 and 21 are less commonly observed.

All EGFR mutations are observed in adenocarcinoma of the lung, although they can also be seen in adenosquamous carcinomas. EGFR mutations are more commonly observed in young female patients with no history of smoking but there can be exceptions to this. EGFR mutations are very rarely observed in pure squamous cell carcinoma of the lung. In patients who develop resistance to EGFR TKIs, secondary mutations in EGFR are observed, the commonest is the T790M activating point mutation in exon 20 [17, 18, 24–29].

4.3 BRAF

BRAF is a proto-oncogene that encodes a serine/threonine protein kinase that is a downstream effector protein of RAS and it transduces the signal through the mitogen-activated protein kinase pathway, which promotes cell proliferation and survival. Phosphorylation of downstream mediators MEK1 and MEK2 occurs on activation of BRAF, which subsequently activates ERK1 and ERK2, which take part in the regulation of growth-regulating proteins such as c-JUN and ELK1. BRAF-activating mutations lead to an increase in the kinase activity that exhibits transforming activity in vitro.

BRAF mutations are most commonly noted in melanoma, and they can also occur in about 3% cases of NSCLC. The mutations seen in NSCLC differ from those in melanoma and colorectal carcinoma. In lung adenocarcinoma, V600E mutations in exon 15 are most commonly seen accounting for 50% of BRAF mutations, which are followed by G469A in exon 11 and D594G in exon 15. In NSCLC BRAF mutations occur either in the kinase domain (such as V600E, D594G, and L596R) or in the G-loop of the activation domain of the gene (such as G465V and G468A). BRAF and EGFR mutations are mutually exclusive. Non-V600E BRAF mutations are observed in current or former smokers, while V600E mutations are more common in female never smokers. BRAF mutations act as an important therapeutic target in NSCLC [14, 21, 30, 31].

4.4 MEK

MEK1 (also known as MAPK1) is a serine–threonine kinase that acts as an important downstream target of RAS activation. MEK1 further activates MAPK2 and MAPK3 that are downstream of BRAF. In lung adenocarcinoma, somatic mutations of MEK1 are reported rarely and they are mostly activating mutation in exon 2 [27, 32].

4.5 Met

MET is located on chromosome 7q21-q31 and acts as a protooncogene that encodes a membrane tyrosine kinase receptor that is also known by the name hepatocyte growth factor receptor. Hepatocyte growth factor binds to its ligand, there occurs a sequence of events which are homodimerization of receptor, activation of kinase, and downstream signaling through PI3K/AKT/RAS/RAF/MEK/MAPK and c-SRC kinase pathways. Gene amplification of MET is observed in NSCLC. MET copy number is increased more commonly in SCC than ADC and is mutually exclusive with KRAS mutations. Amplification of MET results in overexpression of MET protein and thus activation of downstream signaling pathways. MET amplification is a known mechanism of secondary EGFR-TKI resistance. In this scenario, the amplification of MET drives and maintains the PI3K/AKT pathway bypassing the EGFR blockade by TKIs, which suggests concomitant MET inhibition may be a way of overcoming TKI resistance [33–36].

4.6 HER-2

The human epidermal growth factor receptor 2 (HER2/ERBB2) is a part of the ERBB family of receptors which encodes a membrane-bound receptor tyrosine kinase. Unlike other members of ERBB receptors, it does not bind directly to the ligand but can form heterodimers with other ligand-bound members of the receptor family. On activation, there occurs signaling through PI3K, MAPK, and JAK/STAT pathways. HER2 activation is seen in only a few cases of lung cancers with 20% of the case showing overexpression, gene amplification in 2%, and activating mutations in 1.6–4% of NSCLC. HER2 mutations are most commonly observed in adenocarcinoma and this mutation occurs mostly in tumors that are wild type for EGFR and KRAS and they are observed in the female gender, Asian ethnicity, and non-smokers, which is similar to the clinical profile of EGFR mutant tumors [37–41].

4.7 ROS1

ROS1, a proto-oncogene, belongs to receptor tyrosine kinase of the insulin family receptor and is located on chromosome 6q22. The rearrangement was initially described in glioblastoma involving the ROS1-FIG gene fusion.

More recently, ROS1 fusions were identified as potential driver mutations in an NSCLC cell line (HCC78; SLC34A2-ROS1) and an NSCLC patient sample (CD74-ROS1). These fusions result in tyrosine kinase activation, although the details of the downstream signaling transduced by ROS1 fusion are not fully understood yet.

Patients with ROS1 rearrangements are significantly younger, more likely to be never smokers, and overrepresented in the Asian race. Also, ROS-positive lung cancer patients are associated with sensitivity toward TKIs, specifically crizotinib, with a patient demonstrating prompt and durable complete response to therapy [42–44].

4.8 Ret

It is a proto-oncogene that encodes for receptor tyrosine kinase and is located on chromosome 10q11.2. The chromosomal rearrangements involving RET gene and kinesin family 5B (KIF5B) & coiled-coil domain containing-6 (CCDC6) resulting in KIF5B-RET and CCDC6-RET fusion genes have been identified in 70 to 90% and 10 to 25% of lung tumors, respectively.

As a result of chromosomal rearrangements, there is overexpression of RET protein. The RET fusion is found in 1–2% of NSCLC, particularly in younger, non-smoking patients with adenocarcinoma histology, and is associated with increased risk of brain metastases and patients with RET fusions show minimal response to immunotherapy [43–46].

4.9 ALK

ALK encodes for receptor tyrosine kinase. Mutation of the ALK gene is associated with 4% of unselected NSCLC approximately. EML4-ALK fusion gene that is found in a subset of lung cancers occurs because of chromosomal rearrangements forming EML4–ALK fusion gene that is involved in the activation and upregulation of RAS/RAF1/MAP2K1/MAPK1 pathway that is involved in cell proliferation as well as cell survival.

Lung cancers associated with ALK rearrangements are more common in young patients with male dominance who are more commonly non-smokers or light smokers. These tumors show typical histology characterized by the presence of mucin as well as the solid pattern of tumor growth comprising of signet cells in the Western population or acinar growth pattern in Asian patients. They are commonly diagnosed at an advanced stage of clinical presentation. The response rate to chemotherapy as well as the overall survival rate in patients with ALK rearrangement is prompt and comparable [42, 47–50].

4.10 DDR2

The DDR2 gene is a tyrosine kinase receptor, present on the long arm of chromosome 1 (1q23.3). It is involved in cell proliferation, survival, and migration by promoting matrix metalloproteinase expression. DDR2 mutation is associated with 3.8% of cases of squamous cell carcinoma. DDA2 mutations have also been observed in a few cases of NSCLC. It acts as an oncogene and its over expression promotes cell survival and proliferation in SCC lungs [51–53].

4.11 FGFR

FGFR belongs to the receptor tyrosine kinase family and is one of the most promising predictive biomarkers in lung cancer. There is overexpression and gain of function mutation of FGFR in lung cancer. Fibroblast growth factors bind with FGFR causing the activation and upregulation of JAK–STAT/MAPK/PI3K-AKT pathway causing cell proliferation, angiogenesis, differentiation, and survival. Multiple FGFR aberrations are present in Sq-NSCLC tumors—alterations (mutations and fusions), amplification, and mRNA/protein over-expression—but their predictive potential is unclear. FGFR1 amplification is seen in 22% of lung squamous cell carcinoma patients. Mutations are more common in non-smokers than smokers, with more advanced TNM stages. FGF mutations in small-cell carcinoma lung is associated with poor prognosis [54–56].

5. Tumor suppressor genes

5.1 TP53

TP53 (Tumor protein 53) is a tumor suppressor gene located on chromosome 17p13. It encodes a protein containing DNA binding, transcriptional activation, and oligomerization domains. The encoded protein regulates the expression of certain target genes involved in cell cycle arrest, DNA repair, or metabolic changes. It also regulates the expression of genes engaged in promoting growth arrest in the G1 phase or cell death in response to genotoxic stress. P53 is thus known as "the guardian of the genome." P53 prevents the damaged cells from undergoing mitosis. On entering the G2 phase, p53 blocks cells at the G2 checkpoint, by inhibiting the cyclin-dependent kinase required to enter mitosis. This ability of p53 to inhibit cellular proliferation or induce apoptosis is suppressed by the HDM2 protein product. There is proteosome-dependent degradation and downregulation of p53 expression caused by HDM2 protein. Also, p53 itself causes the activation of HDM2 protein by binding directly with HDM2 protein resulting in the upregulation of HDM2. Thus, p53 downregulates its own expression, and as a result of which, p53 levels in normal cells are merely detectable because of this autoregulatory mechanism. Damaged DNA inducesTP53 activation leading to cell cycle arrest by inducing the expression of cyclin-dependent

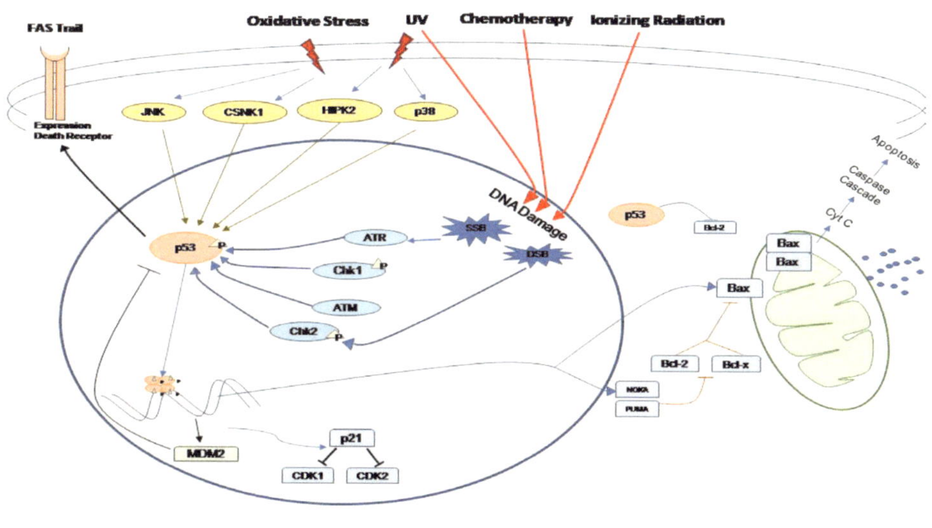

Figure 4.
TP53 pathway.

kinase inhibitors, which may cause DNA repair or apoptosis (**Figure 4**). One of the most common abnormalities noted in lung cancer is the inactivation of TP53 with a hemizygous deletion of 17p13, containing the locus of TP53, which accounts for 90% of mutations of small-cell carcinomas and about 65% of NSCLC. Missense mutations involving TP53 have been known to be associated with 80–100% of small-cell lung carcinomas. In NSCLC mutations or proteins, accumulation has been known to occur more commonly in SCC than in ADC. Also, mutations of TP53 were found in at least 81% of SCCs in a meta-analysis by the cancer genome atlas (TCGA). Exposure to tobacco and smoking has also been noted to be associated with the varied nature of the mutation spectrum as smoking-associated cancers have a higher propensity of G to T transversions compared to G to C transversions due to the presence of polycarbonates associated with tobacco smoke. Also, G to A transitions at CpG dinucleotides are more commonly seen in never smokers. Mutations of EGFR and KRAS can also occur in association with TP53, and also, loss of function mutation of TP53 has been associated with poor response to treatment [57–64].

5.2 LKB1 (STK11)

The LKB1 is a tumor suppressor gene located on chromosome 19p13.3. It was thought to be involved as the causative agent behind Peutz-Jeghers syndrome through a germline-inactivating mutation. LKB1 mutation is typically rare in most types of cancer, except pancreatic cancer and NSCLC. It was found that LKB1 possesses inactivating mutations in NSCLC tumors. Inactivation of LKB1 is known to be more common in adenocarcinomas than in squamous cell carcinomas at a rate of 34 and 19%, respectively. LKB1 in lung cancer may be inhibited by a variety of somatic mutations or deletions that produce truncated proteins causing inactivation of LKB1in about 11–30% of lung ADC. It is thought to be the third commonest genetic aberration in lung ADC after TP53 and KRAS. There are few studies in the literature supporting the association between LKB1 mutations and a history of smoking in men. Also, a correlation with KRAS mutations has been reported [65–67].

5.3 PTEN

PTEN, a tumor suppressor gene, is located on the long arm of chromosome 10 and encodes for lipid and protein phosphatases. This phosphatase causes the dephosphorylation of PIP3 as a result of which there is downregulation in the expression of PI3K/AKT/mTOR signaling pathway. Thus, the loss of function mutation of PTEN results in unrestricted upregulation and activation of signaling pathways causing uncontrolled cell proliferation, resulting in tumor mass. Some lung cancers are associated with PTEN mutations or deletions. PTEN mutations are more common in smokers than non-smokers, present in 10.2% cases of SCC lung as compared to 1.7% cases of adenocarcinoma lung. Overall, PTEN mutations are seen in 5% cases of NSCLC, in which 75% cases of NSCLC show reduced protein expression [68, 69].

5.4 PI3K

The PI3K/mTOR/AKT pathway is an important signal transduction pathway involved in the regulation of cell proliferation, differentiation, survival, adhesion, and motility. Both NSCLC and small-cell carcinoma have been known to be associated with alterations in this pathway. A variety of membrane tyrosine kinase receptors including EGFR, vascular endothelial growth factor receptors, insulin-like growth factor receptors, HER2, and platelet-derived growth factor receptors has been known to activate this pathway. Activation of tyrosine kinase receptors results in the phosphorylation of PIP2 (phosphatidylinositol 4, 5-bisphosphate) to PIP3 (phosphatidyl inositol 3,4,5-triphosphate) with the help of enzymes phospho inositol 3 kinase (PI3K). PI3K and mTOR further cause phosphorylation of PIP3. Downstream regulation of AKT is caused by mTOR, which is a serine/threonine kinase. Activation and upregulation of AKT result in cell proliferation and survival. Also, upregulation of other pathways like RAF/MAPK/RAS results in direct activation of PIP3 [70–73].

6. Therapeutic approach

Targeted drug therapy is recommended for the treatment of lung cancers. It is primarily used to treat non-small-cell lung cancers that constitute 80–85% of lung cancers. It targets the abnormalities in tumor cells without damaging the healthy cells. Biomarker testing is emerging as a tool in targeted therapy for testing patients who have abnormalities in their DNAs, which can be detected after looking for changes in the tumor cells. These changes can be additions, deletions, point mutations, rearrangements, or genetic alterations in the DNA. These changes are targeted in most lung cancer treatments. Targeted therapy is often associated with fewer side effects as they focus on the specific target that is mutated in the cell. These drugs target the pathways involved in lung adenocarcinomas. A number of pathways have been implicated in the causation of lung cancer such as EGFR, PI3K/AKT/mTOR, NTRK/ROS1, and RAS–MAPK, which have been targeted for the treatment purpose. Targeted therapy drugs have now replaced chemotherapy as the first-line treatment, such as EGFR inhibitors erlotinib, gefitinib, PI3K/AKT/mTOR inhibitors everolimus, and NTRK/ROS1 inhibitors entrectinib. These drugs have been found to be clinically beneficial and safer than conventional chemotherapy in the treatment of lung cancer [74, 75].

7. Conclusion

The knowledge of the large genomic data including the role of oncogenes, proto-oncogenes as well as tumor suppressor genes has markedly improved the understanding of the pathogenesis of lung cancers to develop more effective targeted therapies. The recent development in molecular testing technologies has led to the identification of genetic alterations. In addition to the above-mentioned molecular biomarkers, efforts are going on in an extensive manner to identify additional aberrations that can be further explored and used in the targeted therapy of lung cancer. This will further help to improve the available treatment strategies, tailor targeted therapies, and provide newer treatment avenues.

Author details

Shivani Gandhi*, Ishani Gupta, Reetika Menia and Raman Kumar
All India Institute of Medical Sciences, Jammu and Kashmir, India

*Address all correspondence to: dr.shivanigandhi@gmail.com

References

[1] Malik PS, Raina V. Lung cancer: Prevalent trends & emerging concepts. The Indian Journal of Medical Research. 2015;**141**(1):5-7. DOI: 10.4103/0971-5916.154479

[2] Ferlay J, Soerjomataram I, Ervik M, Dikshit R, Eser S, Mathers C, et al. GLOBOCAN 2012 v1.0, Cancer Incidence and Mortality Worldwide: IARC CancerBase No. 11. Lyon, France: International Agency for Research on Cancer; 2013

[3] Indian Council of Medical Research. National Cancer Registry Programme. Three Year Report of Population Based Cancer Registries: 2009-2011. Indian Council of Medical Research; 2013

[4] Inamura K. Lung cancer: Understanding its molecular pathology and the 2015 WHO classification. Frontiers in Oncology. 2017;**7**:193. DOI: 10.3389/fonc.2017.00193

[5] Lindeman NI, Cagle PT, Beasley MB, Chitale DA, Dacic S, Giaccone G, et al. Molecular testing guideline for selection of lung cancer patients for EGFR and ALK tyrosine kinase inhibitors: Guideline from the College of American Pathologists, International Association for the Study of Lung Cancer, and Association for Molecular Pathology. Journal of Thoracic Oncology. 2013;**8**:823-859

[6] Thunnissen E, van der Oord K, den Bakker M. Prognostic and predictive biomarkers in lung cancer. A review. Virchows Archiv. 2014;**464**:347-358

[7] Lynch TJ, Bell DW, Sordella R, Gurubhagavatula S, Okimoto RA, Brannigan BW, et al. Activating mutations in the epidermal growth factor receptor underlying responsiveness of non-small-cell lung cancer to gefitinib. The New England Journal of Medicine. 2004;**350**:2129-2139

[8] Mok TS, Wu YL, Thongprasert S, Yang CH, Chu DT, Saijo N, et al. Gefitinib or carboplatin-paclitaxel in pulmonary adenocarcinoma. The New England Journal of Medicine. 2009;**361**:947-957

[9] Roh MS. Molecular pathology of lung cancer: Current status and future directions. Tuberculosis and Respiratory Diseases (Seoul). 2014;**77**(2):49-54

[10] Ju YS, Lee WC, Shin JY, et al. A transforming KIF5B and RET gene fusion in lung adenocarcinoma revealed from whole-genome and transcriptome sequencing. Genome Research. 2012;**22**:436-445

[11] Kohno T, Ichikawa H, Totoki Y, et al. KIF5B-RET fusions in lung adenocarcinoma. Nature Medicine. 2012;**18**:375-377

[12] Lipson D, Capelletti M, Yelensky R, et al. Identification of new ALK and RET gene fusions from colorectal and lung cancer biopsies. Nature Medicine. 2012;**18**:382-384

[13] Cancer Genome Atlas Research Network. Comprehensive genomic characterization of squamous cell lung cancers. Nature. 2012;**489**:519-525

[14] Downward J. Targeting S signalling pathways in cancer therapy. Nature Reviews. Cancer. 2003;**3**:11-22

[15] Karnoub AE, Weinberg RA. Ras oncogenes: Split personalities. Nature Reviews. Molecular Cell Biology. 2008;**9**:517-531

[16] Bos JL. Ras oncogenes in human cancer: A review. Cancer Research. 1989;**49**:4682-4689

[17] Ding L, Getz G, Wheeler DA, et al. Somatic mutations affect key pathways in lung adenocarcinoma. Nature. 2008;**455**:1069-1075

[18] Yip PY, Yu B, Cooper WA, et al. Patterns of DNA mutations and ALK rearrangement in resected node negative lung adenocarcinoma. Journal of Thoracic Oncology. 2013;**8**:408-414

[19] Riely GJ, Kris MG, Rosenbaum D, et al. Frequency and distinctive spectrum of K S mutations in never smokers with lung adenocarcinoma. Clinical Cancer Research. 2008;**14**:5731-5734

[20] Rodenhuis S, Slebos RJ. Clinical significance of ras oncogene activation in human lung cancer. Cancer Research. 1992;**52**:2665s-2669s

[21] Schmid K, Oehl N, Wrba F, et al. EGFR/KRAS/BRAF mutations in primary lung ADC and corresponding locoregional lymph node metastases. Clinical Cancer Research. 2009;**15**:4554-4560

[22] Subramanian J, Govindan R. Molecular genetics of lung cancer in people who have never smoked. The Lancet Oncology. 2008;**9**:676-682

[23] Linardou H, Dahabreh IJ, Kanaloupiti D, et al. Assessment of somatic k- S mutations as a mechanism associated with resistance to EGFR-targeted agents: A systematic review and meta-analysis of studies in advanced non- small-cell lung cancer and metastatic colorectal cancer. The Lancet Oncology. 2008;**9**:962-972

[24] Inamura K, Ninomiya H, Ishikawa Y, Matsubara O. Is the epidermal growth factor receptor status in lung cancers reflected in clinicopathologic features? Archives of Pathology & Laboratory Medicine. 2010;**134**:66-72

[25] Eberhard DA, Giaccone G, Johnson BE. Biomarkers of response to epidermal growth factor receptor inhibitors in non–small-cell lung cancer working group: Standardization for use in the clinical trial setting. Journal of Clinical Oncology. 2008;**26**:983-994

[26] Liu P, Morrison C, Wang L, et al. Identification of somatic mutations in non-small cell lung carcinomas using whole exome sequencing. Carcinogenesis. 2012;**33**:1270-1276

[27] Kosaka T, Yatabe Y, Endoh H, et al. Mutations of the epidermal growth factor receptor gene in lung cancer: Biological and clinical implications. Cancer Research. 2004;**64**:8919-8923

[28] Shigematsu H, Lin L, Takahashi T, et al. Clinical and biological features associated with epidermal growth factor receptor gene mutations in lung cancers. Journal of the National Cancer Institute. 2005;**97**:339-346

[29] Rekhtman N, Paik PK, Arcila ME, et al. Clarifying the spectrum of driver oncogene mutations in biomarker-verified squamous carcinoma of lung: Lack of EGFR/KRAS and presence of PIK3CA/AKT1 mutations. Clinical Cancer Research. 2012;**18**:1167-1176

[30] Davies H, Bignell GR, Cox C, et al. Mutations of the BRAF gene in human cancer. Nature. 2002;**417**:949-954

[31] Marche IA, Chen TH, Richards WG, et al. Clinical features and outcome of patients with non–small-cell lung cancer harboring BRAF mutations. Journal of Clinical Oncology. 2011;**29**:3574-3579

[32] Marks JL, Gong Y, Chitale D, et al. Novel MEK1 mutation identified by mutational analysis of epidermal growth factor receptor signaling pathway genes in lung adenocarcinoma. Cancer Research. 2008;**68**:5524-5528

[33] Sadiq AA, Salgia R. MET as a possible target for non–small-cell lung cancer. Journal of Clinical Oncology. 2013;**31**:1089-1096

[34] Beau-Faller M, Ruppert AM, Voegeli AC, et al. MET gene copy number in non-small cell lung cancer: Molecular analysis in a targeted tyrosine kinase inhibitor naive cohort. Journal of Thoracic Oncology. 2008;**3**:331-339

[35] Go H, Jeon YK, Park HJ, et al. High MET gene copy number leads to shorter survival in patients with non-small cell lung cancer. Journal of Thoracic Oncology. 2010;**5**:305-313

[36] Engelman JA, Zejnullahu K, Mitsudomi T, et al. MET amplification leads to getinib resistance in lung cancer by activating ERBB3 signaling. Science. 2007;**316**:1039-1043

[37] Tzahar E, Waterman H, Chen X, et al. A hierarchical network for interreceptor interactions determines signal transduction by Neu differentiation factor/neuregulin and epidermal growth factor. Molecular and Cellular Biology. 1996;**16**:5276-5287

[38] Graus-Porta D, Beerli RR, Daly JM, et al. ErbB-2, the preferred heterodimerization partner of all ErbB receptors, is a mediator of lateral signalling. The EMBO Journal. 1997;**16**:1647-1655

[39] Heinmöller P, Gross C, Beyser K, et al. HER2 status in non-small cell lung cancer: Results from patient screening for enrollment to a phase II study of herceptin. Clinical Cancer Research. 2003;**9**:5238-5243

[40] Shigematsu H, Takahashi T, Nomura M, et al. Somatic mutations of the HER2 kinase domain in lung adenocarcinomas. Cancer Research. 2005;**65**:1642-1646

[41] Tomizawa K, Suda K, Onozato R, et al. Prognostic and predictive implications of HER2/ERBB2/neu gene mutations in lung cancers. Lung Cancer. 2011;**74**:139-144

[42] Shaw AT, Yeap BY, Mino-Kenudson M, et al. Clinical features and outcome of patients with non-small-cell lung cancer who harbor EML4-ALK. Journal of Clinical Oncology. 2009;**27**:4247-4253

[43] Bergethon K, Shaw AT, Ou SH, et al. ROS1 rearrangements define a unique molecular class of lung cancers. Journal of Clinical Oncology. 2012;**30**:863-870

[44] Takeuchi K, Soda M, Togashi Y, et al. RET, ROS1 and ALK fusions in lung cancer. Nature Medicine. 2012;**18**:378-381

[45] Drilon A, Lin JJ, Filleron T, et al. Frequency of brain metastases and multikinase inhibitor outcomes in patients with RET-rearranged lung cancers. Journal of Thoracic Oncology. 2018;**13**:1595-1601

[46] Mazieres J, Drilon A, Lusque A, et al. Immune checkpoint inhibitors for patients with advanced lung cancer and oncogenic driver alterations: Results from the IMMUNOTARGET registry. Annals of Oncology. 2019;**30**:1321-1328

[47] Selinger CI, Rogers TM, Russell PA, et al. Testing for ALK rearrangement in lung adenocarcinoma-a multicenter comparison of immunohistochemistry

and fluorescent in situ hybridization. Modern Pathology. 2013;**26**:1545-1553

[48] Rodig SJ, Mino-Kenudson M, Dacic S, et al. Unique clinicopathologic features characterize ALK-rearranged lung adenocarcinoma in the Western population. Clinical Cancer Research. 2009;**15**:5216-5223

[49] Sakairi Y, Nakajima T, Yasufuku K, et al. EML4-ALK fusion gene assessment using metastatic lymph node samples obtained by endobronchial ultrasound-guided transbronchial needle aspiration. Clinical Cancer Research. 2010;**16**:4938-4945

[50] Wong DW, Leung EL, So KK, et al. The EML4-ALK fusion gene is involved in various histologic types of lung cancers from nonsmokers with wild-type EGFR and KRAS. Cancer. 2009;**115**:1723-1733

[51] Ren T, Zhang J, Liu X, Yao L. Increased expression of discoidin domain receptor 2 (DDR2): A novel independent prognostic marker of worse outcome in breast cancer patients. Medical Oncology. 2013;**30**(1):397

[52] Sasaki H, Shitara M, Yokota K, Okuda K, Hikosaka Y, Moriyama S, et al. DDR2 polymorphisms and mRNA expression in lung cancers of Japanese patients. Oncology Letters. 2012;**4**(1):33-37

[53] Fathi Z, Mousavi SAJ, Roudi R, Ghazi F. Distribution of KRAS, DDR2, and TP53 gene mutations in lung cancer: An analysis of Iranian patients. PLoS One. 2018;**13**(7):e0200633. DOI: 10.1371/journal.pone.0200633

[54] Weiss J, Sos ML, Seidel D, Peifer M, Zander T, Heuckmann JM, et al. Frequent and focal FGFR1 amplification associates with therapeutically tractable FGFR1 dependency in squamous cell lung cancer. Science Translational Medicine. 2010;**2**(62):62-93

[55] Li JJ, Yan S, Pan Y, Liu Z, Liu Y, Deng Q, et al. FGFR genes mutation is an independent prognostic factor and associated with lymph node metastasis in squamous non-small cell lung cancer. Cancer Biology & Therapy. 2018;**19**(12):1108-1116. DOI: 10.1080/15384047.2018.1480294

[56] Presta M, Dell'Era P, Mitola S, et al. Fibroblast growth factor/fibroblast growth factor receptor system in angiogenesis. Cytokine & Growth Factor Reviews. 2005;**16**:159-178

[57] Mogi A, Kuwano H. TP53 mutations in non small cell lung cancer. Journal of Biomedicine & Biotechnology. 2011;**2011**:583929

[58] Wistuba II, Berry J, Behrens C, et al. Molecular changes in the bronchial epithelium of patients with small cell lung cancer. Clinical Cancer Research. 2000;**6**:2604-2610

[59] D'Amico D, Carbone D, Mitsudomi T, et al. High frequency of somatically acquired p53 mutations in small-cell lung cancer cell lines and tumors. Oncogene. 1992;**7**:339-346

[60] Tammemagi MC, McLaughlin JR, Bull SB. Meta-analyses of p53 tumor suppressor gene alterations and clinicopathological features in resected lung cancers. Cancer Epidemiology, Biomarkers & Prevention. 1999;**8**:625-634

[61] Husgafvel-Pursiainen K, Boffetta P, Kannio A, et al. p53 mutations and exposure to environmental tobacco smoke in a multicenter study on lung cancer. Cancer Research. 2000;**60**:2906-2911

[62] Takagi Y, Osada H, Kuroishi T, et al. p53 mutations in non-small-cell lung cancers occurring in individuals without a past history of active smoking. British Journal of Cancer. 1998;**77**:1568-1572

[63] Steels E, Paesmans M, Berghmans T, et al. Role of p53 as a prognostic factor for survival in lung cancer: A systematic review of the literature with a meta-analysis. The European Respiratory Journal. 2001;**18**:705-719

[64] Forgacs E, Zochbauer-Muller S, Olah E, Minna JD. Molecular genetic abnormalities in the pathogenesis of human lung cancer. Pathology Oncology Research. 2001;**7**(1):6-13

[65] Koivunen JP, Kim J, Lee J, et al. Mutations in the LKB1 tumour suppressor are frequently detected in tumours from Caucasion but not Asian lung cancer patients. British Journal of Cancer. 2008;**99**:245-252

[66] Matsumoto S, Iwakawa R, Takahashi K, et al. Prevalence and specificity of LKB1 genetic alterations in lung cancers. Oncogene. 2007;**26**:5911-5918

[67] Sanchez-Cespedes M, Parrella P, Esteller M, et al. Inactivation of LKB1/STK11 is a common event in adenocarcinomas of the lung. Cancer Research. 2002;**62**:3659-3662

[68] Cully M, You H, Levine AJ, et al. Beyond PTEN mutations: The PI3Kpathway as an integrator of multiple inputs during tumorigenesis. Nature Reviews. Cancer. 2006;**6**:184-192

[69] Jin G, Kim MJ, Jeon HS, et al. PTEN mutations and relationship to EGFR, ERBB2, KRAS, and TP53 mutations in non-small cell lung cancers. Lung Cancer. 2010;**69**:279-283

[70] Brognard J, Clark AS, Ni Y, et al. Akt/protein kinase B is constitutively active in non-small cell lung cancer cells and promotes cellular survival and resistance to chemotherapy and radiation. Cancer Research. 2001;**61**:3986-3997

[71] Tsurutani J, West KA, Sayyah J, et al. Inhibition of the phosphatidylinositol3-kinase/Akt/mammalian target of rapamycin pathway but not the MEK/ERK pathway attenuates laminin-mediated small cell lung cancer cellular survival and resistance to imatinib mesylate or chemotherapy. Cancer Research. 2005;**65**:8423-8432

[72] Papadimitrakopoulou V. Development of PI3K/AKT/MTOR pathway inhibitors and their application in personalized therapy for non-small-cell lung cancer. Journal of Thoracic Oncology. 2012;**7**:1315-1326

[73] Vivanco I, Sawyers CL. The phosphatidylinositol 3-kinase-AKT pathway inhuman cancer. Nature Reviews. Cancer. 2002;**2**:489-501

[74] Ferlay J, Soerjomataram I, Dikshit R, Eser S, Mathers C, Rebelo M, et al. Cancer incidence and mortality worldwide: Sources, methods and major patterns in GLOBOCAN 2012. International Journal of Cancer. 2015;**136**(5):E359-E386

[75] Fumarola C, Bonelli MA, Petronini PG, Alfieri RR. Targeting PI3K/AKT/mTOR pathway in non small cell lung cancer. Biochemical Pharmacology. 2014;**90**(3):197-207

Chapter 9

Deep Learning-Based Segmentation of Cellular Membranes in Colorectal Immunohistochemical Images

Maisun Mohamed Al-Zorgani, Hassan Ugail, Klaus Pors and Abdullahi Magaji Daudu

Abstract

The segmentation of cellular membranes is essential for getting crucial information in diagnosing several cancers, including lung, breast, colon, gastric cancer, etc. Manual segmentation of cellular membranes is a tedious, time-consuming routine and prone to error and inter-observer variation. So, it is one of the challenges that pathologists face in immunohistochemical (IHC) tissue images. Although automated segmentation of cellular membranes has recently gained considerable attention in digital pathology applications, little research is based on machine learning approaches. Therefore, this study proposes a deep framework for semantic segmenting cellular membranes using an end-to-end trainable Convolutional Neural Network (CNN) based on encoder and decoder architecture with Atreus Spatial Pyramid Pooling (ASPP). The backbone of the encoder depends on the residual architecture. The performance of the proposed framework was evalu ated and compared to other benchmark methods. As a result, we show that the proposed framework exhibits significant potential for cellular membranes segmentation in IHC images.

Keywords: cellular membrane segmentation, immunohistochemistry (IHC) staining images, GLUT-1 protein expression, deep learning approach, Convolutional Neural Network (CNN)

1. Introduction

Immunohistochemistry (IHC) is an efficient staining technique used in pathology to localise a certain antigen in a tissue specimen. Hence, It is now employed in state-of-the-art research to identify specific antigens within a tissue sample from formalin-fixed paraffin-embedded (FFPE) tissue, e.g. in tissue microarrays (TMAs) and 3D dimensional spheroids grown from cells. The cellular membranes segmentation of IHC images is usually required in histopathology to provide more relevant information for diagnosing particular cancers because specific tumour antigens are expressed in certain cancers. Glucose transporter-1 (GLUT-1) is one of the well-known biomarkers bound with the cellular membrane that induces and increases hypoxic conditions in different solid tumours, including breast, prostate, and colorectal cancer [1]. The production of Hypoxia-Inducible Factors (HIFs) proteins in tumour hypoxia regions activates GLUT-1 genes that promote hypoxia [2]. Oxygen gradient, supply and distribution in hypoxic areas lead to the difference in size and extension in all solid tumour regions [3]. Tumour hypoxia is a unique hallmark of cancer due to the difference in oxygen demand and supply, which produces cancer stem cell niche, resistance to therapy (chemotherapy and radiotherapy), immune damping, poor clinical prognosis and genomic instability [3, 4]. Currently, tumour hypoxia is receiving significant attention as the centre for the hallmarks of cancer; this is because of its many characteristics of chemotherapy and radiotherapy resistance and a primary prognostic factor [5]. In clinical practice, assessing the development and spread of hypoxia across solid tumours is an essential routine performed by pathologists to describe the appropriate therapy. In the deep hypoxic environment, It is getting more difficult for chemotherapy and radiotherapy to reach tumour sites. Thus, the need for using hypoxia-activated pro-drugs (HAPs) as targeted therapy is needed.

In recent years, Computer-Aided Diagnosis (CAD) technologies have emerged as one of the potential solutions for histopathological image analysis. The CAD technologies have been used to quantitatively and objectively evaluate IHC biomarkers in a whole tissue slide or a specific region of interest delineated by a pathologist. So, they have been employed to assist histopathologists in some laborious routines, such as visual examination of IHC images for scoring and segmenting the cellular membrane. Thus, the advantages of CAD technologies are avoiding inconsistency in the diagnosis among pathologists, improving the diagnosis quality and reducing the diagnostic time. On the other hand, machine learning-based CAD technologies rely heavily on hand-crafted features that can be significantly prone to feature extractor bias. In addition, relevant domain knowledge is necessary to select the valuable features. Thus, hand-crafted techniques can only deal with some low-level information of images. In contrast, deep learning-based CAD techniques are characterised by; 1) Their ability to extract high-level abstract features from images automatically in a standardised way [6, 7], 2) Their ability to analyse entire slides in detail rather than focusing on a region of interest (ROI) [8], 3) Their ability to learn complex mapping functions directly from the input data and 4) Their ability to avoid personal user bias, as it does not require manual extraction of specific visual features [9]. Hence, they deliver unbiased outcomes for dataset images [9]. So, this work proposes deep learning based-segmentation of the cellular membranes in colorectal IHC images.

The remainder of this chapter is organised as follows. Section 2 presents the related works. Section 3 provides the materials, proposed framework and evaluation indices that are used in this work. Section 4 reports the experimental results from the proposed model. Finally, in Section 5, we discuss analyses of the results and conclude the chapter.

2. Related work

Automated segmentation of cellular membranes has received much attention lately. Various machine learning-based approaches for segmenting the cell membranes in IHC images have been proposed [10–14]. Chang et al. [10] employed the colour channel to extract the morphology, texture and intensity features that then have been utilised to train the support vector machine (SVM) classifier. Tuominen et al. [12] employed conventional machine learning techniques and ImageJ in preparing their ImmunoMembrane web application. Kuo et al. [14] employed a watershed algorithm for nucleus segmentation. But all these algorithms are not up to the performance of deep learning approaches. Therefore, there is a demanding need to employ deep learning approaches, which are advanced machine learning approaches for solving the current issues related to membrane segmentation. Several researchers [15–17] investigated deep learning approaches for cell membranes segmentation. Khameneh et al. [15] employed the SVM classifier to specify ROI and then the deep U-net model for segmenting membrane regions. Saha et al. [16] proposed a long short term memory (LSTM) architecture to detect cell membrane and nucleus. Gaur et al. [17] proposed deep CNN based on the active learning technique for membrane segmentation.

An atrous convolution layer is introduced in deepLab-v1 [18] network to widen the receptive field of view over the input feature maps without a decrease in spatial dimensions and an increase in the number of network parameters. And then, multiple parallel atrous convolutional layers with different dilution rates are proposed in the DeepLab v2 [19] network to segment objects at multiple scales. These layers are known as Atrous Spatial Pyramid Pooling (ASPP) model. After that, the ASPP model is improved in DeepLab v3 [20] to concatenate the image level features, a 1x1 convolution and three 3x3 atrous convolutions with different dilution rates. Encoder-Decoder structure and ASPP model are integrated into Deeplab v3+ [21] for applying the depth-wise separable convolution in both ASPP and Decoder modules. The encoder module reduces the spatial dimensions of the feature maps through the repeated application for the convolution and pooling layers, whilst the decoder module gradually recovers the spatial dimensions by using de-convolution and upsampling layers. Then, skip connections are introduced between the encoder and decoder modules to have sharper segmentation results.

In this work, we propose a trainable CNN based-detector to incorporate encoder, ASPP and decoder. We leveraged the identity mappings proposed by He et al. (2016a, b) in their Residual architectures. So, the encoder part employs the pre-trained ResNet-50 network [22] trained on the ImageNet [23] dataset as the feature extractor. Hence, through the proposed detector, we can overcome the challenges of 1) training the entire network from scratch, 2) the data scarcity problem and its consequences, and 3) over-fitting and poor generation of features. The main contributions of our proposed framework are as follows:

- The proposed detector introduces a new way of deep learning-based semantic segmentation of cell membranes.

- The implementation of the ASPP structure improves the performance of the proposed detector.

- The proposed framework incorporated an encoder-decoder network and dilated/atrous convolutions units to tackle the presence of pooling layers issue that reduces the feature maps dimensions ignore the positional information of objects.

- It is value addition in terms of the main quantification in the existing techniques for segmenting the cellular membrane.

3. Material and evaluation methods

3.1 Image dataset acquisition

We evaluated the proposed detector on real IHC dataset images. Dataset images were acquired from the institute of cancer therapeutics at University of Bradford, United Kingdom. The authors have obtained ethical approval for publication. The images were obtained by immunohistochemistry staining on colorectal cancer adenocarcinoma of human clinical specimens. GLUT-1 and ALDH7A1 prepared the immunohistochemistry staining on HT-29 Tissue Microarray (TMA). The TMA clinical sample slide holds 150 cores and has the number G063 (Biomax.us). These cores represent the whole side of the clinical sample and give a total of 50 cases of colorectal cancer in each whole TMA slide. Whereas 100 cores are colorectal tissues, and 50 cores were either malignant, adjacent tissue to the cancer tissue or normal tissues. The clinical samples were collected from colorectal cancer patients (male and female) in July and August 2019. The IHC images were scanned using an Aperio Digital Pathology Slide Scanners (Aperio AT2) and then captured with ×20 magnification and 200 μm diameter. The whole cores and examples of GLUT-1 expression of IHC colon adenocarcinoma images are shown in **Figures 1** and **2**, respectively.

3.2 Pre-processing of dataset images

In a pre-processing step, there are procedures will be applied to the dataset images as follows;

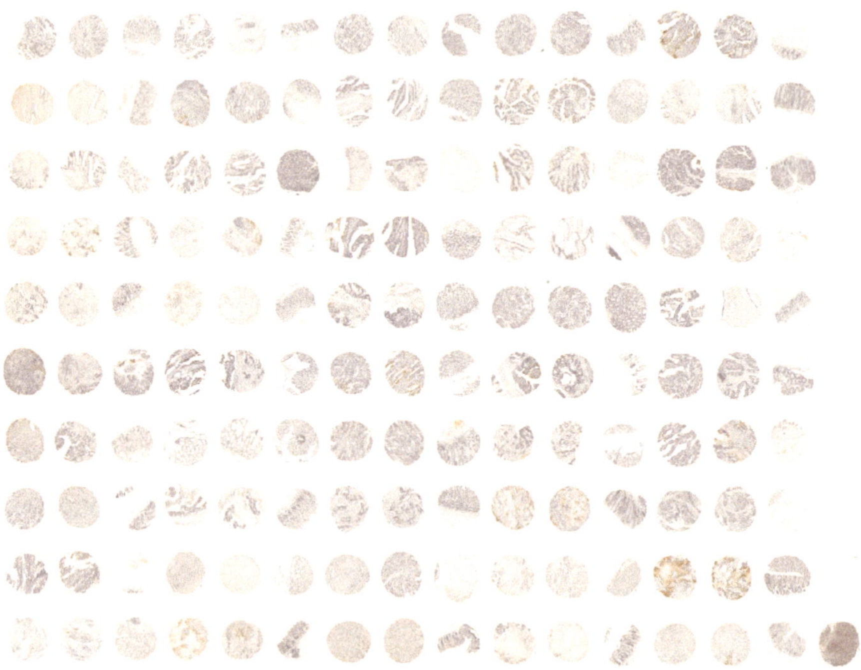

Figure 1.
The G063 TMA slide with 150 cores.

3.3 The evaluation index

The segmentation performance of the proposed detector was assessed by using the popular four evaluation criteria. These criteria use the following metrics; TP, FP, FN and TN denote respectively the number of true positive, false positive, false negative and true negative from all images in the dataset. True positive (TP) is counted as the intersection of a segmented cell membrane with its ground truth; otherwise, it is counted as false positive (FP). False negative (FN) is calculated as the missed parts of the ground truth, and true negative (TN), parts of the image beyond the union segmentation plus ground truth.

3.3.1 Network accuracy metric

This criterion is used to measure a network's ability to segment. It indicates correctly predicted observations against total observations and it is calculated as follows:

$$Accuracy = \frac{TP + TN}{TP + FP + FN + TN} \tag{1}$$

3.3.2 Detection accuracy metric

This criterion is used F1-score metric to measure the detection accuracy of individual cellular membranes. The F1-score is defined by both Precision and Recall metrics. Precision metric indicates the correctly predicted positive observations against total predicted positive observations, whilst Recall metric indicates correctly predicted positive observations against total actual positive observations. F1-score is calculated as follows:

$$F_1Score = \frac{2.Precision.Recall}{Precision + Recall} = \frac{2TP}{2TP + FN + FP} \tag{2}$$

where

$$Precision = \frac{TP}{TP + FP}$$

and

$$Recall = \frac{TP}{TP + FN}$$

3.3.3 Shape similarity metric

This criterion is used Intersection over Union (IoU) also known as Jaccard Similarity Coefficient to compare similarities between segmented cell membranes and their ground truth. The Jaccard index is calculated as follows:

$$Jaccard(IoU) = \frac{TP}{TP + FP + FN} \tag{3}$$

3.3.4 Dice coefficient score

This criterion is used to measure the agreement among segmented cell membranes and their ground truth at object level. The Dice score metric is used the ground set (G) and segment set (S). G; a group of pixels belonging to a ground truth object, and S; a group of pixels belonging to a segmented object. It is utilised to measure similarity between G and S and produces scores between 0 and 1, where 1 indicates perfect segmentation. It is calculated as follows:

$$Dice(G, S) = \frac{2|G \cap S|}{2|G \cap S| + |G| + |S|} \quad (4)$$

3.4 Proposed methodology

We propose a semantic level segmentation of celluar membranes using an end-to-end trainable CNN based on integrates three modules; an encoder, an ASPP, and a decoder. We adapt the ResNet-50 [22] pre-trained on ImageNet [23] as the backbone for encoder module. The inputs are first passed through an extended ResNet50 network, followed by an ASPP module for multi-scale image processing and a decoder module to resize the images to the original input dimensions and produce sharp segmentation results. **Figure 3** shows our architecture and its three main modules. In the following section, there is a brief description of each module:

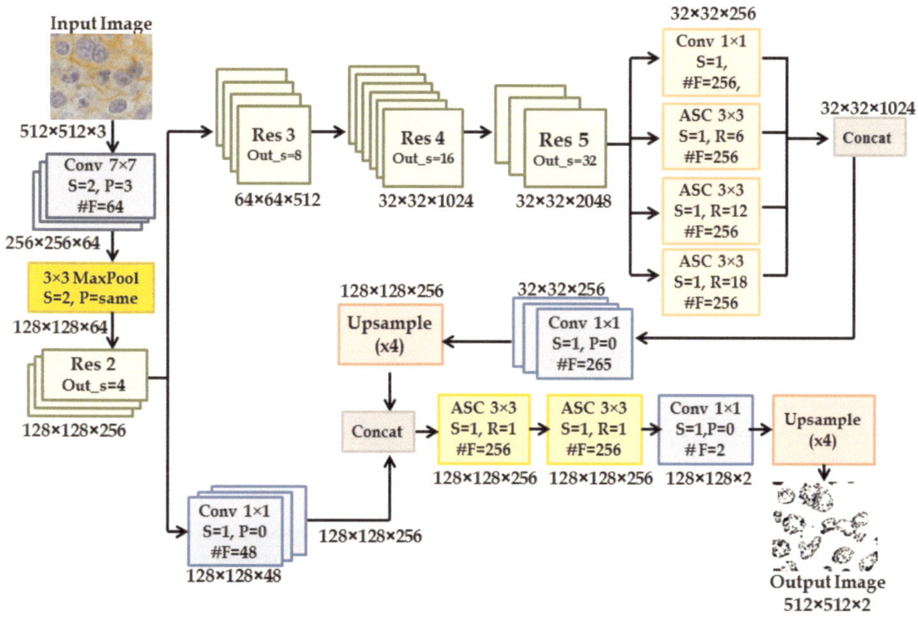

Figure 3.
Show the proposed network architecture, "CONV" represents the convolution blocks that followed by rectified linear unit activation layer (ReLU) and batch normalisation layer (BN); "ASC" represents the atrous separable convolution blocks; "#F" represents the output number of filters for block; "S" represents the stride of all convolutions; P is padding.

3.4.1 Encoder module

It acts as a feature extractor that uses several residual units to reduce the size of an input image. It contains the following blocks;

- An initial block consists of a 7 × 7 convolutional layer with stride 2 and a 3 × 3 max-pooling layer with stride 2, so the output size after this block is reduced by four times (Output stride = 4), and its output is 64 channels.

- Res2 Unit is composed of three blocks (residual error units), all of which are small convolutions of 1 × 1 or 3 × 3, and stride is 1, so the output size after Res2 block is still lower than the original image by four times, the Res2 output is 256 channels.

- Res3 Unit is composed of four blocks, among which the 3 × 3 convolution kernel stride of the first block is 2. Therefore, the output size after Res3 is reduced by eight times relative to the original image (output-stride = 8), and the output of Res3 is 512 channels.

- Res4 Unit is composed of six blocks. The first block is a regular residual block, and the 3 × 3 convolution of the following five blocks use a hole convolution with rate = 2. Therefore, the output size after Res4 is reduced by eight times relative to the original image (output-stride = 8), but the receptive field is reduced by four times close to the original image. The Res4 output is 1024 channels.

- Res5 Unit is composed of three blocks. The first block is the same as Res4, which is a residual with rate = 2. The rate of the 3 × 3 convolution in the last two blocks is 4. Therefore, the output size after Res5 is reduced by eight times relative to the original image (output-stride = 8), but the receptive field is as large as the original image. The Res5 output is 2048 channels.

3.4.2 ASPP module

It applies four parallel Atrous Separable Convolutions (ASC) with different dilation rates; this allows analysing the extracted features at different scales. Whereas, The ASC is a depthwise convolution with atrous convolutions followed by a pointwise convolution. The ASPP output is 1024 channels.

3.4.3 Decoder module

The outputs of the ASPP module are concatenated and passed through a 1 × 1 convolution to reduce the number of channels to 256. This result is upsampled by a factor of four and concatenated with low-level features of the same dimension.

Since the input structure should be aligned with the output structure, thus it is appropriate to share the low-level information, such as edges or shapes, with the higher ones. Then, we apply two 3 × 3 ASCs and, finally, a 1 × 1 convolution with two-channel, so that a binary mask is obtained. This result is upsampled by a factor of four to recover the original size of the image.

4. Experiment and results

In this section, we describe our experiment, analyse the experimental results obtained and then compare the obtained results with the other networks results produced for the same purpose.

4.1 Setup the experiment

The experiment was implemented in MATLAB R2020a on a PC with Intel⊗R, Dual-Core i7–7700 at 3.60 GHz CPU, 64 GB RAM, and NVIDIA GeForce GTX.

1070 GPU. The experiment was carried out using our IHC dataset images as follows;

- The augmented training dataset images were divided randomly into training set 80% (x images) and test set 20% (y images).
- The network is constructed by initialising the weights from a pre-trained ResNet50 model.
- The proposed network was trained by tuning hyperparameters as shown in **Table 1**.

4.2 Results analysis

4.2.1 Traing Progress analysis

The evaluation of proposed detector accuracy and loss function over training time on our IHC dataset images is shown in **Figure 4**. After each training epoch, the accuracy and the loss function were calculated on the training and validation sets to

Hyperparameter	Value
Optimizer	SGDM
LearnRateSchedule	'piecewise'
LearnRateDropPeriod	10
LearnRateDropFactor	0.3
Momentum	0.9
InitialLearnRate	0.001
L2Regularization	0.005
MaxEpochs	30
MiniBatchSize	8
Shuffle	'every-epoch'
ValidationPatience	10
ValidationFrequency	1 per epoch

Table 1.
Hyperparameter.

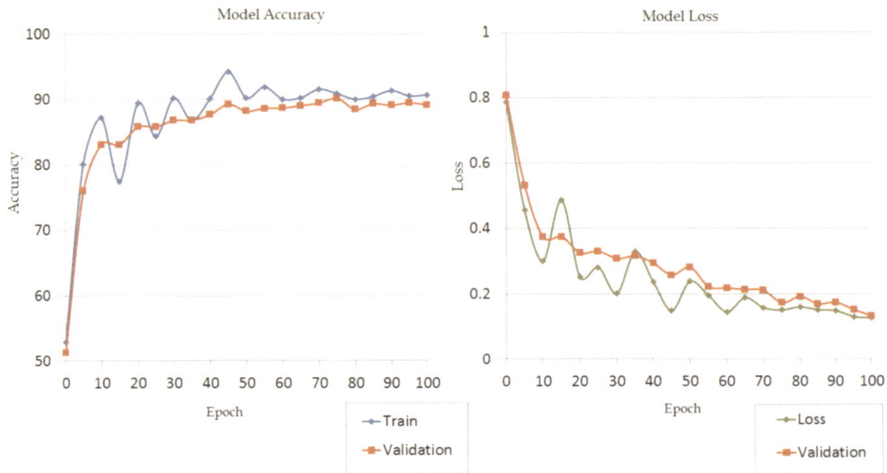

Figure 4.
The training, loss and validation values over the training time.

observe its ability to generalise and avoid overfitting. Throughout the training period, there were raised in the performance in the training set, which corresponded to a decrease in loss value. This behaviour is because the model is still learned to be able to generalise well; however, when the model is able to generalise, the validation loss fluctuates with close to the training loss. As shown in **Figure 4**, the proposed detector converges in the training process through the first 40 epochs, and there are wide fluctuations in performance in the training set, which correspond to fluctuations in loss value. This is expected behaviour during the first epochs of training since the model is still unstable; however, when the model stabilises, the training loss becomes steady with a slight variation close to the validation loss.

4.2.2 Performance analysis

A 2×2 confusion matrix was used to represent the prediction results of the cellular membranes. The matrix was built on two rows and two columns: membranes and non-membranes representing the classes. The 2×2 normalised confusion matrix is shown in **Figure 5**. To statistically analyse the behaviour of our detector at the pixel level, we calculated metrics from the test set using equations; 1, 2 and 3, as reported in **Table 2**. Whereas Dice-Coefficient was calculated at object level using eq. 4.

4.2.3 Comparative analysis

To our knowledge, there are few works that employed a deep learning models to segment cell membranes in IHC images. Hence, to validate our detector and to compare its performance with the state of the art segmentation methods, we first implemented some the public pre-trained models including FCN-8 [29], U-Net [30] and SegNet [31]. The comparative analysis of our detector against the other networks is reported in **Table 3**. When comparing the results produced by our detector with others, we derive that the proposed detector achieved good performance metrics. We get high performance than the popular networks; SegNet, U-Net and FCN-8. At pixel-level, it achieved an F-score value of 0.910. At the object level, it achieved a Dice score value of 0.829.

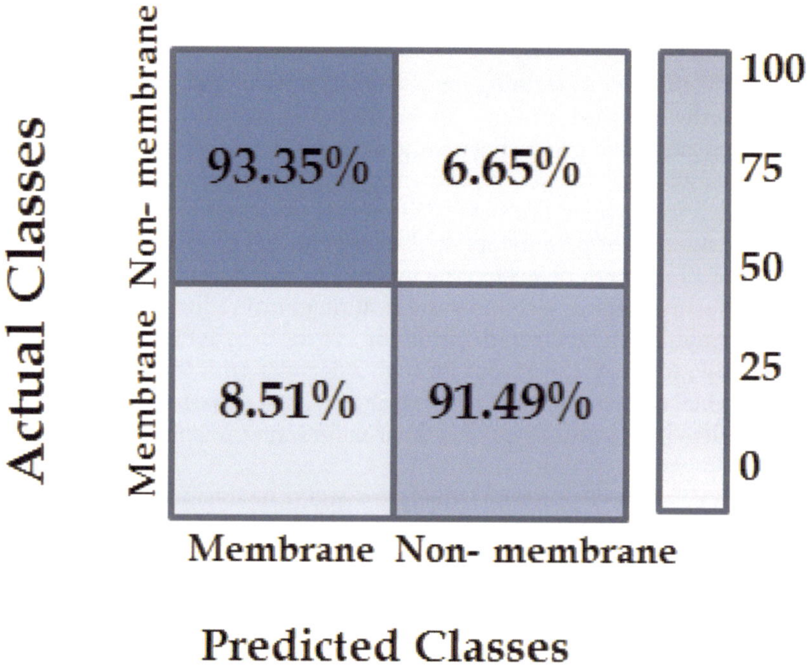

Figure 5.
Normalised confusion matrix for proposed detector.

Metrics	Proposed Detector
Accuracy	0.9227
Recall	0.9335
Precision	0.8874
F_1-score	0.9099
IoU	0.8347
Dice Index	0.829

Table 2.
The statistical metrics of our detector.

Deep model	F1 Score
Eycke et al. [32]	0.844
SegNet	0.858
U-Net	0.862
FCN-8	0.783
Proposed Detector	0.910

Table 3.
Comparative analysis of different models on the IHC dataset.

5. Conclusions

Although the number of training images in our IHC dataset was small, it is observed from the obtained results in these experiments that the proposed detector has significantly achieved promising results in semantic segmentation. This is due to its architecture, which employs the following; firstly, it uses atrous/dilated convolution layers as a way to widen the field of view over the input feature maps without increasing the number of parameters. It also uses the ASPP module to deal with the different scales problem of objects in the image. Furthermore, It uses an encoder-decoder architecture. Hence it reduces the resulting output dimensions through passing multiple convolution layers with strides of 1 or more to avoid pooling layers in the network. Finally, it passes the output through a decoder with learnable parameters to regain the original dimensions. For this reason, we have chosen this architecture for the proposed detector to segment the cellular membranes of colorectal IHC images semantically.

In conclusion, we have presented an end-to-end trainable deep neural network to tackle the problem of cellular membranes in colorectal IHC images. The proposed architecture has achieved a good performance compared with other methods. Hence, the proposed detector is able to objectively and automatically detect glands, thus easing the burden of pathologists.

Conflict of interest

The authors declare that they have no conflict of interest.

Author details

Maisun Mohamed Al-Zorgani[1*], Hassan Ugail[1], Klaus Pors[2] and Abdullahi Magaji Dauda[2]

1 Faculty of Engineering and Informatics, School of Media, Design and Technology, University of Bradford, Bradford, UK

2 Institute of Cancer Therapeutics, University of Bradford, UK

*Address all correspondence to: maisunalzorgani@yahoo.com

References

[1] Huizing FJ, Hoeben BA, Franssen GM, Boerman OC, Heskamp S, Bussink J. Quantitative imaging of the hypoxia-related marker CAIX in head and neck squamous cell carcinoma xenograft models. ACS Publications, Molecular pharmaceutics. 2018;**16**(2): 701-708

[2] Meier V, Guscetti F, Roos M, Ohlerth S, Pruschy M, Rohrer Bley C. Hypoxia-related marker GLUT 1, CAIX, proliferative index and microvessel density in canine oral malignant neoplasia, public library of science San Francisco, CA USA. PLoS One. 2016; **11**(2):e0149993

[3] Bhandari V, Hoey C, Liu LY, Lalonde E, Ray J, Livingstone J, et al. Molecular landmarks of tumor hypoxia across cancer types. Nature Publishing Group, Nature genetics. 2019;**51**(2): 308-318

[4] Zhao S, Yu W, Ukon N, Tan C, Nishijima KI, Shimizu Y, et al. Elimination of tumor hypoxia by eribulin demonstrated by 18 F-FMISO hypoxia imaging in human tumor xenograft models, Springer Open. EJNMMI Research. 2019;**9**(1): 1-10

[5] Mirabello V, Cortezon-Tamarit F, Pascu SI. Oxygen sensing, hypoxia tracing and in vivo imaging with functional metalloprobes for the early detection of non-communicable diseases. Frontiers in Chemistry. 2018, 2018;**6**:27

[6] Yosinski J, Clune J, Bengio Y, Lipson H. How transferable are features in deep neural networks? In: Proceedings of the 27th International Conference on Neural Information Processing Systems. Vol. 2. 2014. pp. 3320-3328

[7] Litjens G, Kooi T, Bejnordi BE, Setio AAA, Ciompi F, et al. A survey on deep learning in medical image analysis. Elsevier journal of medical image analysis. 2017;**42**:60-88

[8] Shah M, Wang D, Rubadue C, Suster D, Beck A. Deep learning assessment of tumor proliferation in breast cancer histological images. In: 2017 IEEE International Conference on Bioinformatics and Biomedicine (BIBM). 2017. pp. 600-603

[9] Ravishankar H, Sudhakar P, Venkataramani R, Thiruvenkadam S, Annangi P. Understanding the mechanisms of deep transfer learning for medical images. In: Deep Learning and Data Labeling for Medical Applications. Springer; 2016. pp. 188-196

[10] Chang C-Y, Huang Y-C, Ko C-C. Automatic analysis of HER-2/neu immunohistochemistry in breast cancer. In: Proc. Third International Conference on Innovations in Bio-Inspired Computing and Applications. 2012. pp. 297-300

[11] Anja B, Mikkel E, Giedrius L, Soren N, Michael G, Hansen Johan D, et al. Digital image analysis of membrane connectivity is a robust measure of HER2 immunostains. Breast Cancer Research and Treatment. 2012;**132**(1):41-49

[12] Tuominen VJ, Tolonen TT, Isola J. Immuno membrane: A publicly available web application for digital image analysis of HER2 immunohistochemistry. Histopathology. 2012;**60**(5):758-767

[13] Ficarra E, Di Cataldo S, Acquaviva A, Macii E. Automated segmentation of cells with IHC membrane staining. IEEE Transactions

on Biomedical Engineering. 2011;**58**(5): 1429-1429

[14] Yung-Lung K, Chien-Chuan K, Lai J-Y. Automated assessment in HER-2/neu immunohistochemical expression of breast cancer. In: Proc. International Symposium on Computer, Communication, Control and Automation (3CA). 2010. pp. 585-588

[15] Khameneh FD, Razavi S, Kamasak M. Automated segmentation of cell membranes to evaluate HER2 status in whole slide images using a modified deep learning network. Computers in Biology and Medicine. 2019;**110**:164-174

[16] Saha M, Chakraborty C. Her2Net: A deep framework for semantic segmentation and classification of cell membranes and nuclei in breast cancer evaluation. IEEE Transactions on Image Processing. 2018;**27**(5):2189-2200

[17] Gaur U, Kourakis M, Newman-Smith E, Smith W, Manjunath BS. Membrane segmentation via active learning with deep networks. In: Proc. IEEE International Conference on Image Processing (ICIP). 2016. pp. 1943-1947

[18] Chen L-C, Papandreou G, Kokkinos I, Murphy K, Yuille AL. Semantic image segmentation with deep convolutional nets and fully connected CRFs. IEEE Transactions on Pattern Analysis and Machine Intelligence. 2018; **40**:834-848

[19] Chen L-C, Papandreou G, Kokkinos I, Murphy K, Yuille AL. Deeplab: Semantic image segmentation with deep convolutional nets, atrous convolution, and fully connected crfs. IEEE Transactions on Pattern Analysis and Machine Intelligence. 2018;**40**:834-848

[20] Chen L-C, Papandreou G, Schroff F, Adam H. Rethinking atrous convolution for semantic image segmentation. arXiv. 2017

[21] Chen L-C, Zhu Y, Papandreou G, Schroff F, Adam H. Encoder-decoder with Atrous separable convolution for semantic image segmentation. In: Proceedings of the European Conference on Computer Vision (ECCV 2018), Munich, Germany, 8–14 September 2018. 2018. pp. 833-851

[22] He K, Zhang X, Ren S, Sun J. Deep residual learning for image recognition. In: Proceedings of the IEEE Conference on Computer Vision and Pattern Recognition (CVPR), Las Vegas, NV, USA, 27–30 June 2016. 2016. pp. 770-778

[23] Russakovsky O, Deng J, Su H, Krause J, Satheesh S, Ma S, et al. Imagenet large scale visual recognition challenge. International Journal of Computer Vision. 2015;**115**:211-252

[24] Ruifrok AC, Johnston DA, et al. Quantification of histochemical staining by color deconvolution. Analytical and Quantitative Cytology and Histology. 2001;**23**(4):291-299

[25] Bayramoglu N, Heikkila J. Transfer learning for cell nuclei classification in histopathology images. In: European Conference on Computer Vision. Springer; 2016. pp. 532-539

[26] Mormont R, Geurts P, Maree R. Comparison of deep transfer learning strategies for digital pathology. In: Proc. IEEE Conference on Computer Vision and Pattern Recognition Workshops. 2018. pp. 2262-2271

[27] Miko-lajczyk A, Grochowski M. Data augmentation for improving deep learning in image classification problem. In: 2018 International Interdisciplinary PhD Workshop (IIPhDW). 2018. pp. 117-122

[28] Shorten C, Khoshgoftaar TM. A survey on image data augmentation for deep learning, springer. J. Big Data. 2019;**6**:60

[29] Long J, Shelhamer E, Darrell T. Fully convolutional networks for semantic segmentation. In: Proceedings of the IEEE Conference on Computer Vision and Pattern Recognition, Boston, MA, USA, 7–12 June 2015. 2015. pp. 3431-3440

[30] Ronneberger O, Fischer P, Brox T. U-net: Convolutional networks for biomedical image segmentation. In: Proceedings of the International Conference on Medical Image Computing and Computer-Assisted Intervention (MICCAI 2015), Munich, Germany, 5–9 October 2015. Vol. 9351. 2015. pp. 234-241

[31] Badrinarayanan V, Kendall A, Cipolla R. Segnet: A deep convolutional encoder-decoder architecture for image segmentation. IEEE Transactions on Pattern Analysis and Machine Intelligence. 2017;**39**:2481-2495

[32] Van Eycke Y-R, Cedric B, Laurine V, Olivier D, Isabelle S, Christine D. Segmentation of glandular epithelium in colorectal tumours to automatically compartmentalise IHC biomarker quantification: A deep learning approach. Medical Image Analysis. 2018; **49**:35-45

Section 3

Molecular Cytopathology

Chapter 10

Cytological Evaluation

Natsuko Mizutani

Abstract

The fact that the human body is composed of cells was demonstrated by Dr. Hooke in 1665, and modern cytology was initiated by Dr. Papanicolaou in 1928. In 1943, Papanicolaou published "Diagnosis of Uterine Cancer by Vaginal Cytology," which is the basis of current cytodiagnostics. There are several types of materials used in cytological diagnosis, each with different methods of specimen preparation and determination. The advantages of some specimen collection methods are that they are less invasive to the body and provide quick determination results. However, correct results cannot be obtained unless the specimen is prepared correctly. In recent years, various methods have been developed with the advancement of imaging tests, the spread of genetic testing, and the spread of artificial intelligence (AI). Liquid-based cytology (LBC) has become widespread, especially in gynecology. It has also become possible to test for human papillomavirus (HPV), which is closely related to cervical cancer, using the same materials. An automated screening system based on a database of morphological characteristics of atypical/tumor cells has also been developed.

Keywords: Papanicolaou's classification, genetic testing, automated screening system, cytology, cervical cancer

1. Introduction

Cytodiagnostics began in 1928 when modern cytology was commenced by Dr. Papanicolaou and was initially recognized for its usefulness as a diagnostic method for cervical cancer (see **Figure 1**) [1]. The examination of smears by Dr. Papanicolaou is one of the most important historical achievements in screening methods for the prevention of disease and cancer. It has been used as a screening test for uterine cancer since 1950. The test is straightforward and practical from a technical perspective and utilizes the simple scientific observation that malignant cells have abnormal nuclear morphology that can be distinguished from benign cells [2–4]. The International Academy of Gynecological Cytology (IAC), which was founded in 1957 and originated from the Japan Gynecological Cytology Discussion Group, was established in Japan in response to the International Academy of Gynecological Cytology (IAGC).

The Japanese Society of Clinical Cytology is a professional society that promotes academic research in clinical cytology and cytodiagnostics and the application of its results to practical clinical practice. Its origins date back to 1961.

Later, in line with advances in other fields of science, the IAC was renamed the International Academy of Cytology in 1961. In 1962, it was joined in Japan with the

IntechOpen

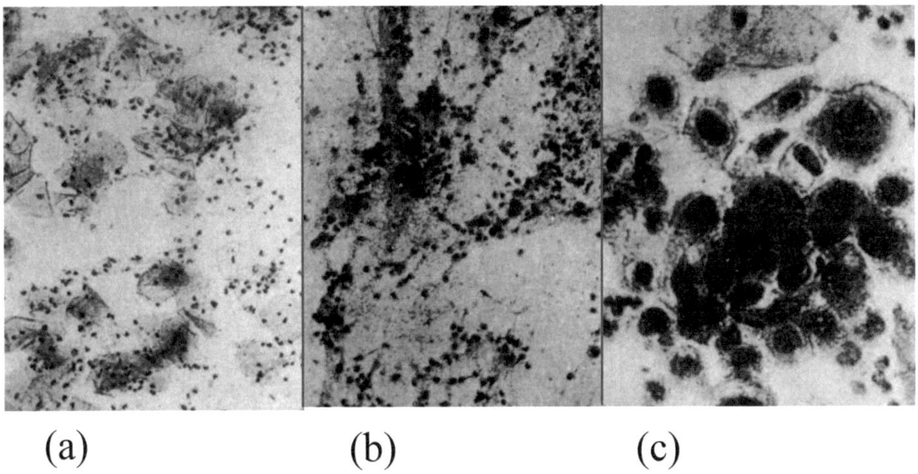

Figure 1.
Gynecological cytology by Dr. Papanicolaou. (a) Normal. (b) Inflammation. (c) Carcinoma. (a) a moderate number of inflammatory cells are seen in the background, and superficial-to-medium squamous epithelium is present. The patient is presumed to be an adult female. (b) A strong inflammatory background is present. (c) The cells differ in enlargement from (a) and (b), but have nuclei that are large and show shape irregularities. Quoted from reference [1], partially modified. George N. Papanicolaou. M.D, New Cancer Diagnosis, The Third Race Betterment Conference, Battle Greek. Michigan. January 2-6. 1928. And published in the proceedings of the Conference the same year.

Tokyo Cytodiagnosis Study Group and others to be known as the Japanese Society of Clinical Cytology.

Since the early 2000s, the academic content of this society has covered numerous fields, including gynecology, surgery, internal medicine, pathology, dentistry, and especially cancer diagnosis. Notably, it is valuable as a means of cancer screening and is used for cervical, uterine, lung, and breast cancer screening. Among these, with its long history, cervical cancer screening has achieved significant results for reducing disease mortality. The Papanicolaou classification was used as a criterion (see **Table 1**). Cells are classified according to their morphological changes from benign (normal or near-normal cells) to malignant (cancerous cells). The Papanicolaou classification, which has five levels from Class I (no abnormality) to Class V (malignant), has been widely used in gynecological cytology because it is easy to compare with histological diagnosis and is common and convenient for other organs.

Class	Comments
I	No abnormal cells
II	Abnormal or abnormal cells present, but no malignant findings
III	Abnormal cells suspected of being malignant are found, but they cannot be determined to be malignant
IIIb	Abnormal cells strongly suspected of being malignant are found, but cannot be determined as malignant
IV	Abnormal cells with strong suspicion of malignancy are observed
V	Recognize cells that can be determined to be malignant

Table 1.
Papanicolaou's classification from the Japanese Society of Clinical Cytology based on gynecology.

DOI: http://dx.doi.org/10.5772/intechopen.109886

Papanicolaou classifications I–V were established in cytology in Japan as the main classification method. Together with the Japanese grouping of the gastrointestinal tract, it supports an easy understanding of the stages of cancer. This classification was believed to be universal and unchanging, and thus, it was perplexing that "overseas, papers written using the Papanicolaou classification are not accepted." Twenty years ago, the Washington Post reported on the low rate of positive cytological diagnoses in the USA using the Papanicolaou classification, and this led to the establishment of the Bethesda system (see **Table 2**) [5–11].

Therefore, why the positive diagnosis rate was so low with the Papanicolaou classification became a question. Various theories exist, including that the specimens were of poor quality, there was an insufficient number of cells smeared, and fixation or staining was not performed properly. Therefore, emphasis was placed on whether enough cells had been collected, whether fixation was adequate, and whether the specimens had been prepared appropriately.

Cytology results are ultimately a judgment based on the individual cytological image obtained. A proper judgment cannot be made if an insufficient amount of sample was collected, thus demonstrating that a necessary quantity must be obtained. This suggests that without proper sampling, accurate determination is not possible. The following section describes the types of collection material and critical points and precautions for specimen preparation. This is very important for a correct assessment.

It has been revised in various ways, and now, some 60 years later, current gynecological cytology is undergoing further changes. Liquefied cytology, which was introduced in Japan later than in Western countries, is becoming more widespread. It is now possible to perform human papillomavirus (HPV) testing on samples taken at the same time [12–15]. This is the time when the efforts for the early detection and treatment of cervical cancer are relevant in terms of cytological diagnosis tests. Furthermore, automatic screening has been initiated.

Cytological tests are now being actively considered not only for cell morphology diagnosis, but also for the introduction of new technologies. These include molecular cytological research on genetic mutations during tumorigenesis and abnormal expression of oncogenes, automated cell diagnosis, and telecytology as part of telemedicine.

2. Materials for cytology determination and evaluation and notes on specimen preparation

Cytodiagnosis is a test that involves the observation of cell images taken from a patient to determine the benign/malignant nature of the cells obtained, among other things.

Cytodiagnosis can be performed by collecting cells in body fluids, such as sputum, urine, pleural fluid, or ascites, or through cell collection with a needle or rubbing with a brush. Depending on the method used to collect the cells, it is classified as exfoliative cytology, puncture aspiration cytology, abrasion cytology, or imprint cytology.

2.1 Exfoliative cytology

Cells spontaneously detach from tissue, often into liquid, such as sputum, urine, milk, pleural fluid, and ascites. The obtained cytogram is often accompanied by

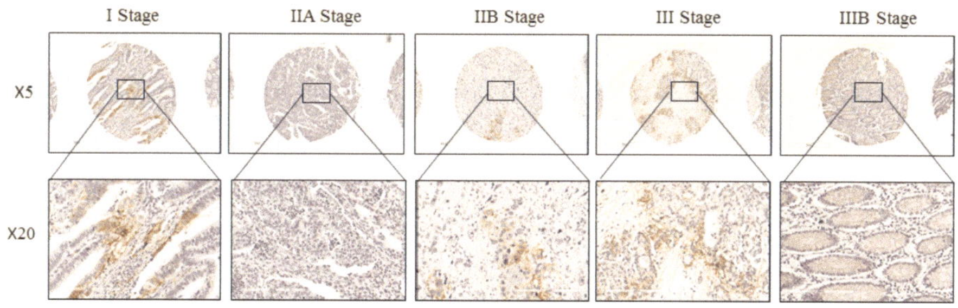

Figure 2.
Examples of GLUT-1 expression at different stages of IHC colon adenocarcinoma images; magnification of upper panel is ×5 and bottom panel is ×20.

3.2.1 Derivation of dataset images

We derived dataset images by hand-picking the ROI from TMA cores that comprised the most representative cells membrane stained. At first, we ran Aperio AT2 program and then selected the ROI regions at a (5× magnification) low resolution. We captured the images from the ROI regions with 20× magnification. A total of 400 IHC images were extracted with size 512 × 512 pixel and then stored in jpeg compression format.

3.2.2 Annotation of dataset images

Two trained pathologists manually annotated the cellular membranes of IHC images according to the proportion of Glut-1 and ALDH7A1 staining. The ground truth images are generated in MATLAB R2020a environment.

3.2.3 Stain normalisation of dataset images

In order to highlight the diaminobenzidine (DAB) stain regions of reactive membranes in the IHC images, we utilised a colour normalisation method described in [24].

3.2.4 Partition of dataset images

We split the dataset images randomly into 80% training set (320 images) and 20% testing set (80 images). The testing set does not utilise for training our proposed detector.

3.2.5 Augmentation of dataset images

Data augmentation is an essential step to generate additional artificial training images by using some transformations for increasing the deep network performance [25, 26]. In this work, we augmented the training images and their ground truth images of our IHC dataset by rotating them with angles of 90, 180 and 270 degrees and then flipping in the horizontal and vertical direction. We chose the rotate and flip transformations to enlarge the training images without affecting the quality of input images [27] and thus avoid the features poorly generalisation and over-fitting problems [28].

Specimen type
Indicate conventional smear (Pap smear), liquid-based preparation (Pap test) vs other
Specimen adequacy
• *Satisfactory for evaluation (describe presence or absence of endocervical/transformation zone component and any other quality indicators, e.g., partially obscuring blood, inflammation, etc.)*
• Unsatisfactory for evaluation (*specify reason*)
○ Specimen rejected/not processed (*specify reason*)
○ Specimen processed and examined, but unsatisfactory for evaluation of epithelial abnormality because of (*specify reason*)
General categorization (optional)
• Negative for intraepithelial lesion or malignancy
• *Other: see Interpretation/Result (e.g., endometrial cells in a woman aged ≥ 45 years)*
• Epithelial cell abnormality: see Interpretation/Result (*specify* "squamous" *or* "glandular," *as appropriate)*
Interpretation/result
Negative for Intraepithelial Lesion or Malignancy
(*When there is no cellular evidence of neoplasia, state this in the General Categorization above and/or in the Interpretation/Result section of the report—whether or not there are organisms or other non-neoplastic findings*)
Non-Neoplastic Findings (optional to report)
Non-neoplastic cellular variations
○ Squamous metaplasia
○ Keratotic changes
○ Tubal metaplasia
○ Atrophy
○ Pregnancy-associated changes
Reactive cellular changes associated with:
■ Inflammation (includes typical repair)
○ Lymphocytic (follicular) cervicitis
■ Radiation
■ Intrauterine contraceptive device (IUD)
Glandular cells status posthysterectomy
Organisms
Trichomonas vaginalis
Fungal organisms morphologically consistent with *Candida* spp.
Shift in flora suggestive of bacterial vaginosis
Bacteria morphologically consistent with *Actinomyces* spp.
Cellular changes consistent with herpes simplex virus
Cellular changes consistent with cytomegalovirus
Other
○ *Endometrial cells (in a woman aged ≥ 45 years)*

(Also specify if "negative for squamous intraepithelial lesion")
Epithelial Cell Abnormalities
Squamous Cell
• Atypical squamous cells
○ Of undetermined significance (ASC-US)
○ Cannot exclude HSIL (ASC-H)
• Low-grade squamous intraepithelial lesion (LSIL)
(Encompassing: HPV/mild dysplasia/CIN-1)
• High-grade squamous intraepithelial lesion (HSIL)
(Encompassing: moderate and severe dysplasia, CIS; CIN-2 and CIN-3)
○ With features suspicious for invasion *(if invasion is suspected)*
• Squamous cell carcinoma
Glandular cell
• Atypical
○ Endocervical cells (NOS *or specify in comments*)
○ Endometrial cells (NOS *or specify in comments*)
○ Glandular cells (NOS *or specify in comments*)
• Atypical
○ Endocervical cells, favor neoplastic
○ Glandular cells, favor neoplastic
• Endocervical adenocarcinoma *in situ*
• Adenocarcinoma
○ Endocervical
○ Endometrial
○ Extrauterine
○ Not otherwise specified (NOS)
Other Malignant Neoplasms (specify)
Adjunctive testing
Provide a brief description of the test method(s) and report the result so that it is easily understood by the clinician
Computer-assisted interpretation of cervical cytology
If case examined by an automated device, specify the device and result
Educational notes and comments appended to cytology reports (optional)
Suggestions should be concise and consistent with clinical follow-up guidelines published by professional organizations (references to relevant publications may be included)
Abbreviation: CIN, cervical intraepithelial neoplasia; CIS, carcinoma *in situ*; HPV, human papillomavirus; NOS, not otherwise specified; Pap, Papanicolaou.
Source: Reprinted from [5].

Table 2.
The 2014 Bethesda system.

degeneration. Care must be taken to consider this part of the image when making a decision. However, there is little burden on the patient, such as pain.

2.2 Abrasion cytology

Cells are collected by rubbing the surface of the tissue in the cervix and bronchi. Cell images should be dried without ethanol fixation as soon as possible after the smear.

2.3 Imprint cytology

Cells are collected by rubbing tissue taken from biopsies or surgery onto a glass slide. As with abrasion cytology, fixation is required immediately after the smear. Care should also be taken not to spoil lymph nodes or undifferentiated tumors if they are suspected.

2.4 Puncture aspiration cytology

The needle test is used to collect lesions from areas under the skin, such as the mammary glands, thyroid gland, and lymph nodes. Fresh cells are obtained, and care must be taken to ensure that the smear and preparation of the specimen are performed as close as possible to recapitulate the situation *in vivo*. Introducing artifacts will prevent correct assessment and diagnosis.

Approximately 10–15 years ago, there was a debate in the Japanese domestic cytological society about the smear method for mammary gland puncture aspiration cytology. The author believes that the smear should be blown at an angle and fixed as it is (see **Figure 2**). At that time, there was an opinion within the academic society that lightly fitting two glass slides together was the correct approach. However, when a trace amount of liquid component is placed between the glass slides, it is technically impossible to lightly align them because of the surface tension, ruining the precious sample.

The author had a bitter experience in understanding this, as shown in **Figures 3** and **4**. These are cases in which the smears are made by matching the glass and destroying the cells; thus, a definitive diagnosis cannot be made. At an academic conference in Japan, several researchers stated that a thick smear is not good because it does not allow the staining solution to enter the smear. For example, if a specimen is cancer, the tumor is a manifestation of a fast cell proliferation rate and high cell density. Adding an artifact to force the stain to cover the tumor in its entirety would destroy the structure of the finalized cell population and result in misdiagnosis. Thus, staining cytology specimens should not be mistaken for paintings.

At symposiums and other meetings of academic societies in Japan, the results were not determined, and the tests were subsequently performed using the chosen approach of each institution. As a result, since around 2015, the rate of positive diagnosis has declined, especially for puncture aspiration cytology of the mammary gland. Guidelines for surgical and treatment methods also indicated tissue biopsy using a thick biopsy needle as the mainstream approach, while preoperative testing for hormone receptors, HER2 sensitivity, and Ki-67 index became the standard [16–18].

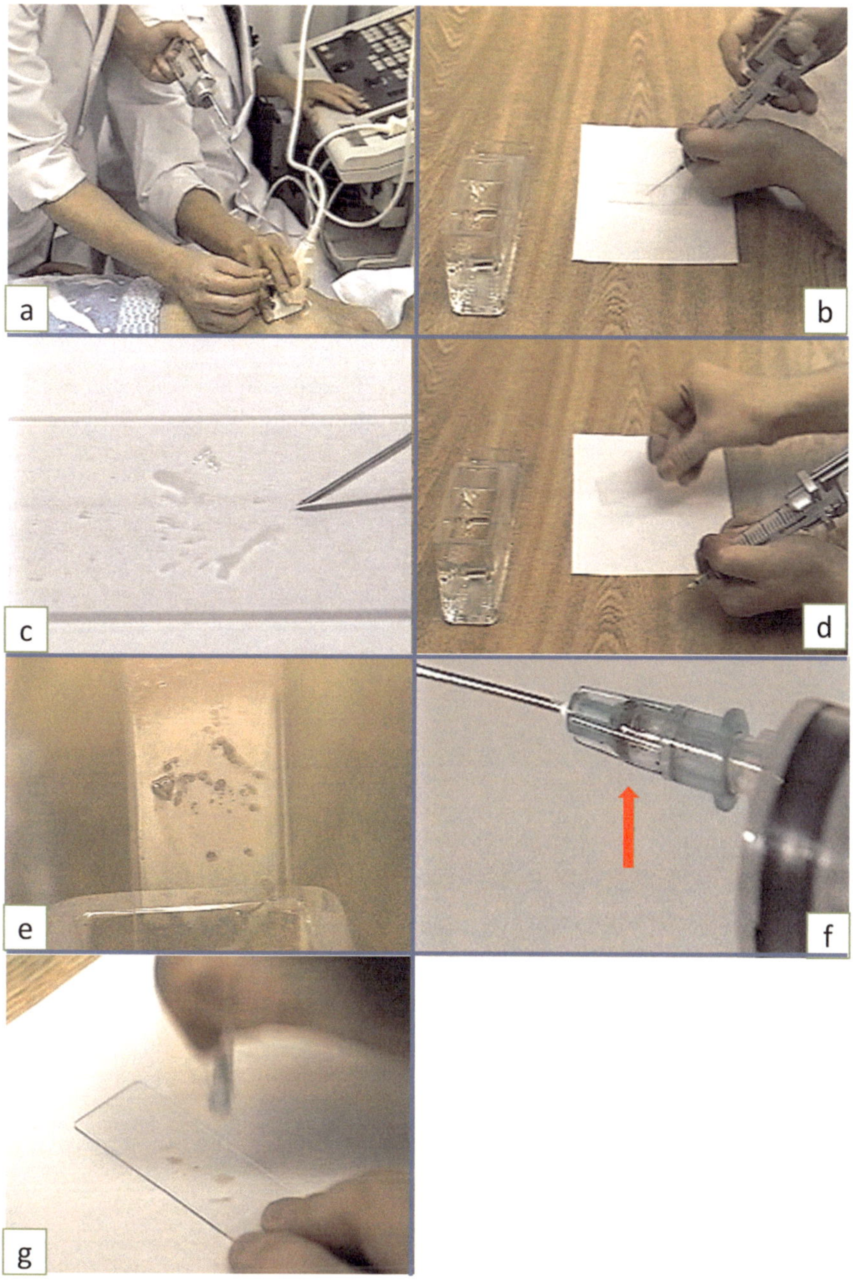

Figure 2.
Standard correct method of fine needle aspiration cytology. (excerpt from an educational video provided by AstraZeneca). (a) this is performed to confirm that the needle is definitely inside the tumor and is done with ultrasound guidance. When the needle tip enters the target site (inside the tumor) aspirate for about 1 minute. Keep the pistol primed (do not scatter cancer cells in the needle). Rotate the needle and gently move it back and forth to push the tumor cells into the needle. Insert, and always return suction when removing the needle. (b) Angle the tip of the needle about 40° and lightly push. Blow onto a glass slide. (c) Point the cut surface of the needle point slightly diagonally instead of straight down. When sprayed, the cells are dispersed almost evenly. (d) Spray the smeared slide glass as it is quickly fixed in alcohol. (e) When remove the alcohol, if it is smeared to the extent shown here, then it is generally okay. (f) Sometimes cells remain at the base of the needle. (g) If this occurs, cap the needle upside down on a slide glass and hit strongly.

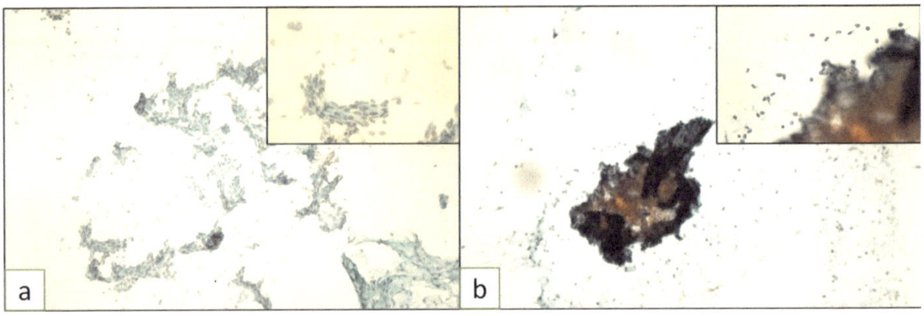

Figure 3.
Fibroadenoma. (a) Laminated glass smear method. (b) Spray smear method. (a) Reported as class III because the cells collapsed due to rubbing together and could not be accurately determined. (b) The bilayered structure of myoepithelial and glandular cells is clear because the cells are not broken.

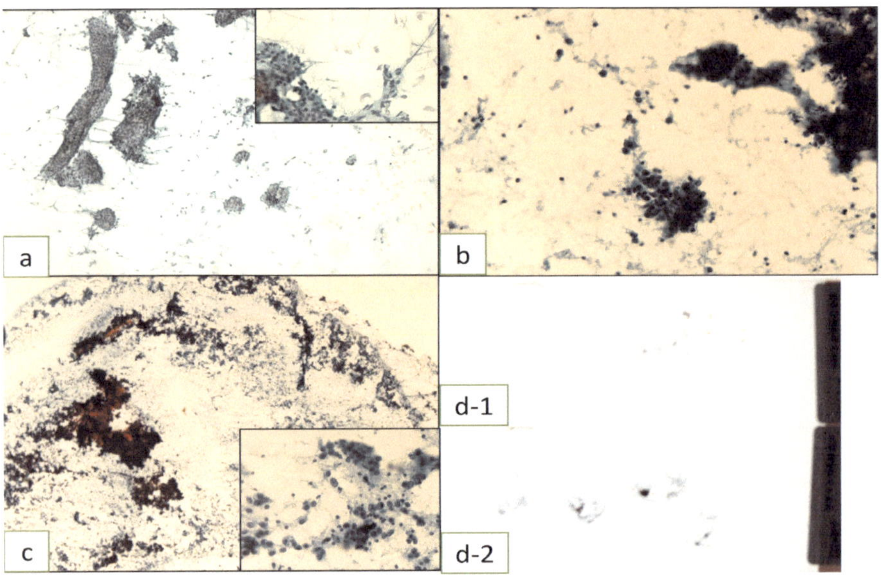

Figure 4.
Ductal carcinoma. (a) Laminated glass smear method. (b) Spray smear method. (c) Smashing smears. (d) Macroscopic image of slide specimen: (d-1) use of the spray smear method; (d-2) use of smashing smears. (a) the individual cells are stretched by the effects of rubbing together. (b, c) the cancer cells have not collapsed. The stacked structure is also preserved.

We hope that the time will come when puncture aspiration cytology will be actively utilized for the follow-up of benign lesions, such as fibroadenomas.

Pancreatic cancer is among the most lethal cancers worldwide because of the limited availability of techniques for the early detection of signs and symptoms. Ultrasound-guided pancreatic puncture aspiration is now also actively performed in some major hospitals [19, 20]. In some hospital facilities, cytological examinations and tissue biopsies are performed together. As the author noted [21], both tests have their own advantages and disadvantages. Unlike tissue biopsy, cytology allows specimens to be obtained from background findings. In the preparation of the tissue specimen, the

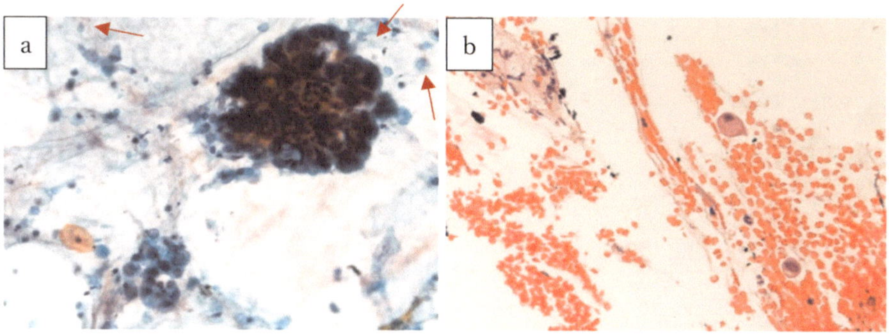

Figure 5.
Adenocarcinoma of the pancreas. (a) Cytology, class V. necrotic material was obtained in the background indicated by the red arrows (). (b) Histology, no malignancy. Only red blood cells and histiocytes were observed in the background. Source: Excerpted from ref. [21], partially modified.

background findings are the parts that are removed by roughing the paraffin block [21]. The presence of cystic or necrotic material in the specimen is a very important diagnostic finding (see **Figure 5**).

2.5 Cell block specimens

Traditionally, cell block specimens have been used when fibrin precipitation has caused cells to adhere to each other and clump together, making smears on glass slides impossible. Sometimes, useful findings can be obtained when the clumped material is used for specimen preparation in the same way as tissue fragments [22–24]. Therefore, immunostaining has recently become increasingly necessary. The reasons for this are the emergence of cancers of unknown primary origin and the widespread use of antibodies for immunostaining.

More recently, when the only symptom is fluid accumulation in the body cavity, such as pleural or ascites fluid, this has been diagnosed as cancer on cytological examination. However, imaging findings of the surrounding organs are not abnormal. Therefore, cell block specimens are prepared from the remaining smear sediment; then, immunostaining is performed to deduce the primary tumor (see **Figure 6**). Based on this, an increasing number of centers are processing specimens with the aim of preparing cell blocks from the outset. Body cavity fluid, which is collected in large quantities, is useful because it tends to have surplus sediment.

Specifically, this process uses disposable tubes made of soft material, as shown in **Figure 7**. Samples are rotated faster than normal centrifugation (3000 rpm, 5 min); then, the supernatant is removed and fixing solution (15% neutral buffered formalin) is added. The sample is left to fix for approximately one day. The specimen is then cut with scissors as shown in the diagram, placed in an embedding cassette, and processed in an automatic embedding machine. Specimens are then prepared in the same way as normal tissue specimens. Ideally, during paraffin embedding, the sediment is picked up with tweezers from inside this tube and embedded directly into the embedding dish, but thin sections can also be made by embedding the entire Japanese tube. An alternative method is to use collodion. The use of sodium alginate has also been considered but should be avoided because it has been reported that sodium alginate may cause some antibodies to become unstained in rare cases.

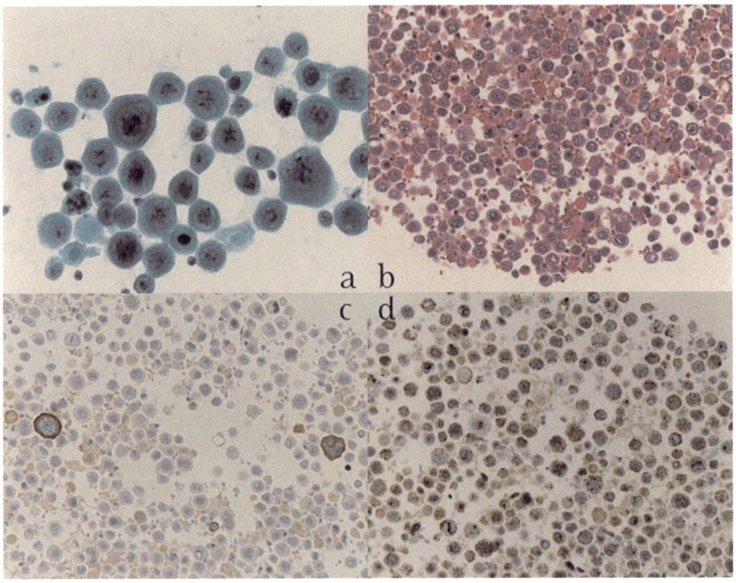

Figure 6.
Microscopic findings for lung adenocarcinoma case. (a) Cytological findings (Papanicolaou). (b) Cell block findings (hematoxylin and eosin). (c) Cell block findings (immunohistochemistry for CEA). (d) Cell block findings (immunohistochemistry for ADC cocktail (TTF-1 and Napsin A)). Excerpt from ref. [24], partially modified.

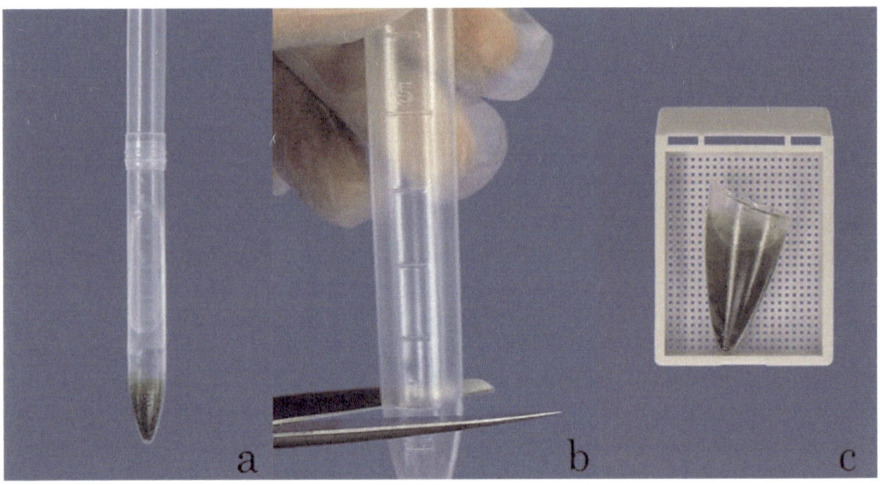

Figure 7.
The cell block producing method. (a) Sample is fixed with 15% formalin solution in tube. (b) Cut the tip of the disposable tube using scissors. (c) The tip of a tube is placed in a cassette. Excerpt from ref. [24], partially modified.

3. Methods introduced in recent years

3.1 ThinPrep integrated imager system mirror inspection support system

In Japan, the cervical cancer screening uptake rate is lower than in Europe and the USA. In addition to improving the uptake rate, training cytologists for screening have become an issue [25–27]. In Europe and the USA, the introduction of liquid-based cytology (LBC) and automatic screening support devices with artificial intelligence (AI) has been progressing to support the high cervical cancer screening uptake rate. Such automatic screening support devices are expected to become widespread in Japan in the future. When one hears the term "automated screening support system,"

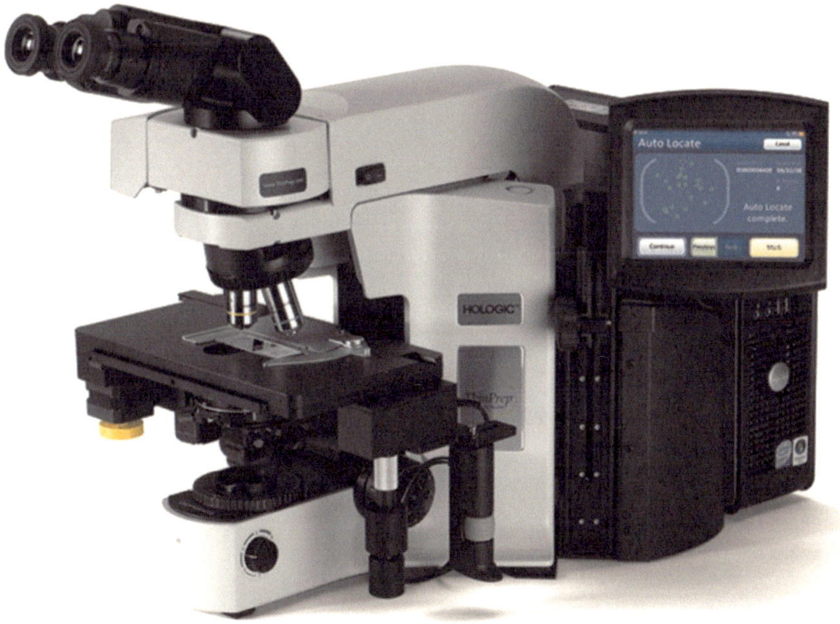

Figure 8.
ThinPrep® integrated imager. Marketing authorization number; 13B1X10179001003.

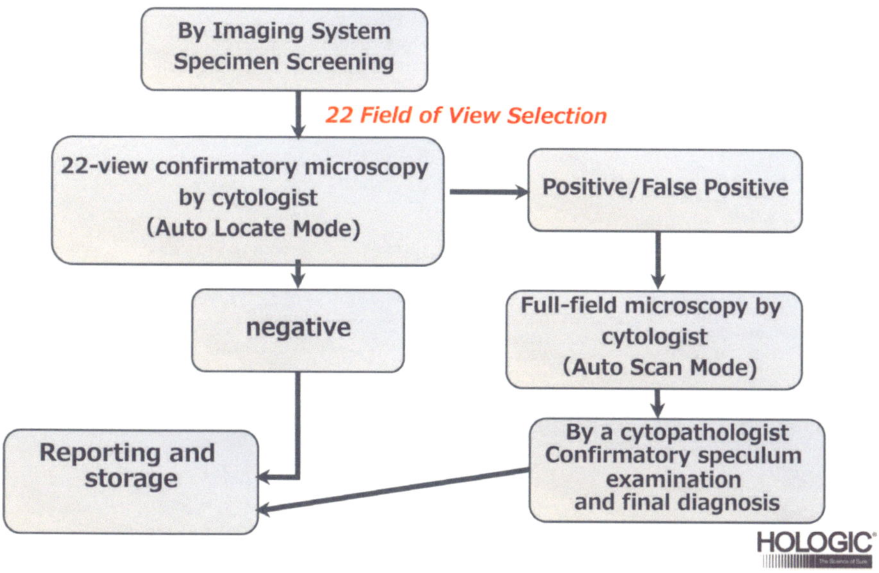

Figure 9.
ThinPrep® imaging system workflow.

one may wonder if it is safe. However, when a cytotechnologist performs the screening, it is undertaken by a human, which entails the risk of oversight and other issues. The concept of this system is to avoid overlooking high-grade squamous intraepithelial lesion (HSIL) lesions.

The system performs two ThinPrep smears for each case. One of them is stained using ThinPrep stain, a staining solution that differs from the usual Papanicolaou stain. The ThinPrep-stained specimens are then set in the machine in advance and

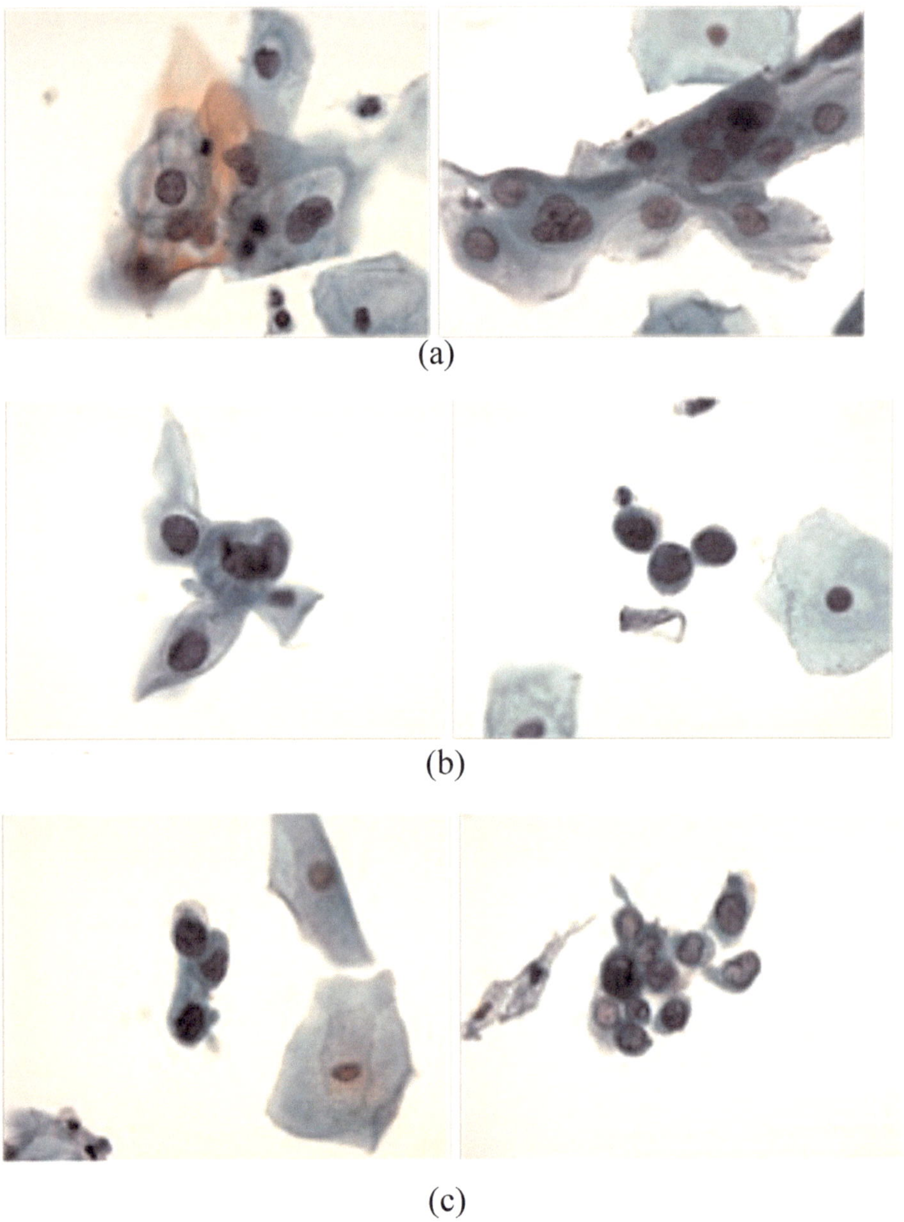

Figure 10.
Manual screening vs. integrated imager screening (I2 screening). (a) M screening: LSIL histology: HSIL/CIN3. (b) I2 screening: HSIL histology: HSIL/CIN3. (c) M screening: Lost histology: HSIL/CIN.

read through, and 22 areas that need to be checked again are selected. These areas are checked with the cytologist using the special microscope shown in **Figure 8** to make a final determination (see **Figure 9**).

This machine (special microscope) shown in **Figure 10** is available from Hologic. A comparison of actual cytologist specimens (M-microscopy) and I2-microscopy (machine) is also shown (see **Table 3**).

ThinPrep-stained specimens appear very dark compared with the normal Papanicolaou stains. However, many of the cells with some atypia have increased chromatin, so they are not likely to be observable by eye unless they are stained somewhat darkly.

The machine then identifies atypical cells at a certain percentage of sensitivity without tiring, unlike humans. In the near future, Japan's aging population is expected to become a serious issue, and this and other factors will increase the need to rely on machines.

However, the author believes that this system would not be effective unless we can make an accurate judgment by looking at the cells presented by this special

			Histology				
			LSIL	**HSIL**			
		Negative	**CIN1**	**CIN2**	**CIN3**	**Adeno**	**Total**
M screening	ASC-US	3	16		2		21
	LSIL		22	3	1		26
	ASC-H		1		3		4
	HSIL		1	2	2		5
	Adeno					2	2
	Total		40	5	8	2	58
I2 screening	ASC-US	2	11				13
	LSIL		28	2			30
	ASC-H	1			5		6
	HSIL		1	3	3		7
	Adeno					2	2
	Total	3	40	5	8	2	58

Agreement rate with tissue diagnosis: LSIL.
M screening: 95.0%.
I2 screening: 97.5%.
Agreement rate with tissue diagnosis: HSIL or higher.
M screening: 60.0%
I2 screening: 86.6% ← *26.6% up!*

Notes)
M screening: Manual screening.
I2 screening: Integrated Imager screening.
Quoted from reference [26], partially modified.
Materials from department of Pathology, Osaka Police Hospital and Hologic, Inc.

Table 3.
Comparison of M screening and I2 screening with Histology.

microscope. It may be meaningless unless the cytologist has the skills to make accurate judgments when presented with several fields of view.

Although Hologic's system requires the preparation of LBC specimens, other companies have developed and marketed systems that allow the use of conventional smears. However, it is assumed that it is quite difficult to create a database based on the conventional method. The system is actually being used by a major testing company, and it is assumed that a considerable number of specimen images are being compiled into a database before it can be used in the current system.

3.2 Combination with HPV testing

HPV testing can now be performed on the same vial from which the LBC specimen is taken for the purpose of cytological diagnosis testing. HPV detection reagents are available from Qiagen, Roche, and BD [28–30]. This seems to be an excellent system for the early detection of dysplastic lesions and the eradication of cervical cancer from both the polymerase chain reaction data and the morphology on the cytogram. In addition, HPV vaccination, which had been on the decline because of adverse reactions, has been actively resumed in Japan.

4. Conclusion

A century has passed since Dr. Papanicolaou began his cytology research. Many cytotechnologists and cytology specialists have played a central role in performing various studies from all sides with the aim of achieving accurate diagnosis. As a result, various meaningful methods have been developed. However, some fields have declined discussions and have become divided and ambiguous. Furthermore, the emergence of AI may cause cytotechnologists to lose their jobs. However, in hindsight, cytology is being effectively used, which is possibly unique to the modern area. This is considered to be proof that cytological diagnosis is highly evaluated worldwide.

Conflict of interest

The author declares no conflict of interest.

Author details

Natsuko Mizutani
Faculty of Health Sciences, Department of Medical Technology, Kyorin University, Japan

*Address all correspondence to: natsuko@ks.kyorin-u.ac.jp

References

[1] Third Race Betterment Conference. Battle Creek, Michigan; 1928

[2] Papanicolaou GN. A new procedure for staining vaginal smears. Science. 1942;**95**:438-439

[3] Diamantis A, Magiorkinis E, Koutselini H. 50 years after the death of George Nicholas Papanicolaou (1883–1962): Evaluation of his scientific work. Acta Medico-Historica Adriatica. 2014; **12**:181-188

[4] Smith ER, George SH, Kobetz E, Xu X-X. New biological research and understanding of Papanicolaou's test. Diagnostic Cytopathology. 2018;**46**: 507-515

[5] Nayar R, Wilbur DC. The pap test and Bethesda 2014. Cancer Cytopathology. 2015;**123**:271-281

[6] Solomon D. Foreword. In: Nayar R, Wilbur DC, editors. The Bethesda System for Reporting Cervical Cytology. Definitions, Criteria, and Explanatory Notes. 3rd ed. Springer; 2015

[7] The 1988 Bethesda system for reporting cervical/vaginal cytologic diagnoses. National Cancer Institute Workshop. JAMA. 1989;**262**:931-934

[8] Kurman RJ, Solomon D, editors. The Bethesda System for Reporting Cervical/ Vaginal Cytologic Diagnoses. Definitions, Criteria, and Explanatory Notes for Terminology and Specimen Adequacy. New York, NY: Springer-Verlag; 1994

[9] Solomon D, Davey D, Kurman R, Moriarty A, O'Connor D, Prey M, et al. Forum group members; Bethesda 2001 workshop. The Bethesda system 2001: Terminology for reporting the results of cervical cytology. Journal of the American Medical Association. 2002; **287**:2114-2119

[10] Solomon D, Nayar R, editors. The Bethesda system for reporting cervical cytology. In: Definitions, Criteria, and Explanatory Notes. 2nd ed. New York, NY: Springer-Verlag; 2004

[11] Sherman ME, Dasgupta A, Schiffman M, Nayar R, Solomon D. The Bethesda Interobserver reproducibility study (BIRST): A web-based assessment of the Bethesda 2001 system for classifying cervical cytology. Cancer Cytopathology. 2007;**111**:15-25

[12] Agorastos T, Chatzistamatiou K, Katsamagkas T, Koliopoulos G, Daponte A, Constantinidis T, et al. Primary screening for cervical cancer based on high-risk human papillomavirus (HPV) detection and HPV 16 and HPV 18 genotyping, in comparison to cytology. PLoS One. 2015; **10**:e0119755

[13] Belinson JL, Qiao YL, Pretorius RG, Zhang WH, Rong SD, Huang MN, et al. Shanxi Province cervical cancer screening study II: Self-sampling for high-risk human papillomavirus compared to direct sampling for human papillomavirus and liquid based cervical cytology. International Journal of Gynecological Cancer. 2003;**13**:819-826

[14] Belinson SE, Wulan N, Li R, Zhang W, Rong X, Zhu Y, et al. SNIPER: A novel assay for human papillomavirus testing among women in Guizhou, China. International Journal of Gynecology Cancer. 2010;**20**:1006-1010

[15] Bigras G, de Marval F. The probability for a pap test to be abnormal

is directly proportional to HPV viral load: Results from a Swiss study comparing HPV testing and liquid-based cytology to detect cervical cancer precursors in 13,842 women. British Journal of Cancer. 2005;**93**:575-581

[16] National Comprehensive Cancer Network Clinical Practice Guidelines in Oncology. Breast Cancer. 1997–2009. (Referenced with permission from The NCCN Clinical Practice Guidelines in Oncology® for Guidelines 1997–2009. © National Comprehensive Cancer Network, Inc. 2010. All rights reserved. To view the most recent and complete version of the guideline, go online to www.nccn.org.)

[17] Institute NC. Breast Cancer Treatment–for Health Professionals (PDQ®) [Internet]. 2015. [Accessed: December 02, 2015]

[18] Hill DA, Friend S, Lomo L, Wiggins C, Barry M, Prossnitz E, et al. Breast cancer survival, survival disparities, and guideline-based treatment. Breast Cancer Research and Treatment. 2018;**170**:405-414. DOI: 10.1007/s10549-018-4761-7

[19] Hewitt MJ, McPhall MJ, Possamai L, Char A, Vlavianos P, Monahan KJ. EUS-guided FNA for diagnosis of solid pancreatic neoplasms: A meta-analysis. Gastrointestinal Endoscopy. 2012;**75**: 319-331

[20] Gonzalo-Marin J, Vila JJ, Perez-Miranda M. Role of endoscopic ultrasound in the diagnosis of pancreatic cancer. World Journal of Gastrointestinal Oncology. 2014;**6**:360-368

[21] Mizutani N, Mochizuki M, Toki M. Assessment of preoperative pancreatic biopsy, cytological/histological review of cell-block-specimens obtained by endoscopic ultrasound-guided fine-needle aspiration. Diagnostic Cytopathology. 2020;**48**:408-413

[22] Krogerus LA, Andersson LC. A simple method for the preparation of paraffin-embedded cell blocks from fine needle aspirates, effusions and brushings. Acta Cytologica. 1988;**3**(2): 585-587

[23] Kung IT, Chan SK, Lo ES. Application of the immunoperoxidase technique to cell block preparations from fine needle aspirates. Acta Cytologica. 1990;**34**:297-303

[24] Nobuhiro R, Shibata J, Kobayashi G, Wakimoto M, Sasaki N. Evaluation of cytologic analysis of alimentary system and effusion fluid specimens by simple cell block method. Medical Technology. 2015;**64**:196-201

[25] ThinPrep Integrated Imager Operating Manual 2014. Hologic, Inc.; 2014

[26] Kaneda A, Yasuoka H, Gunji Y, Fukuda S, Aoki H, Shimada K, et al. Benefits of the ThinPrep integrated imager for cervical cytology. Journal of the Japanese Society of Clinical Cytology. 2019;**58**:189-195

[27] Biscotti CV, Dawson AW, Dziura B, Galup L, Kabawat S. Assisted primary screening using the automated ThinPrep imaging system. American Journal of Clinical Pathology. 2005;**123**:281-287

[28] Nance KV. Evolution of pap testing at a community hospital: A ten year experience. Diagnostic Cytopathology. 2007;**35**:148-153

[29] McDonough SH, Giachetti C, Yang Y, Kolk DP, Billyard E, Mimms L. High throughput assay for the simultaneous or separate detection of human immunodeficiency virus (HIV)

and hepatitis type C virus (HCV). Transfusion Medicine and Hemotherapy. 1998;**25**:164-169

[30] IARC (WHO) IARC Handbooks of Cancer Prevention. Vol. 10. IARC Press; 2005